Practice the HOBET®!

Health Occupations Basic Entrance Test

Practice Test Questions

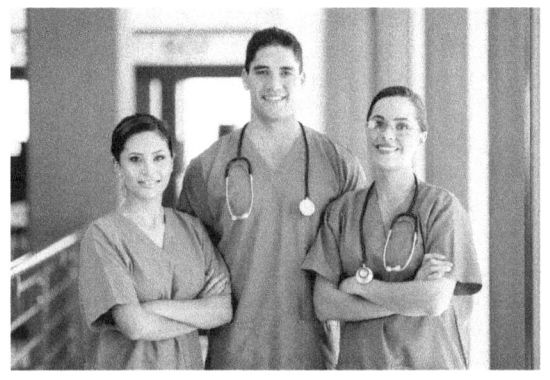

We strongly recommend that students check with exam providers for up-to-date information regarding test content.

ISBN-13: 978-1482533514

ISBN-10: 1482533510

Version 6.5 April 2015

Published by
Blue Butterfly Books
BC Canada
Printed in the USA

Team Members for this publication

Editor: Sheila M. Hynes, MES York, BA (Hons)
Contributor: Dr. C. Gregory
Contributor: Elizabeta Petrovic MSc (Mathematics)
Contributor: Kelley O'Malley BA (English)

Feedback

We welcome your feedback. Email us at feedback@test-preparation.ca with your comments and suggestions. We carefully review all suggestions and often incorporate reader suggestions into upcoming versions. As a Print on Demand Publisher, we update our products frequently.

Contents

Getting Started

CONGRATULATIONS! By deciding to take the Health Occupations Basic Entrance Test (HOBET®) Exam, you have taken the first step toward a great future! Of course, there is no point in taking this important examination unless you intend to do your very best to earn the highest grade you possibly can. That means getting yourself organized and discovering the best approaches, methods and strategies to master the material. Yes, that will require real effort and dedication on your part but if you are willing to focus your energy and devote the study time necessary, before you know it you will be opening that letter of acceptance to the school of your dreams.

We know that taking on a new endeavour can be a little scary, and it is easy to feel unsure of where to begin. That's where we come in. This study guide is designed to help you improve your test-taking skills, show you a few tricks of the trade and increase both your competency and confidence.

The Test of Essential Academic Skills Exam

Content areas for the HOBET® are: Reading, Math, Science and English.

Reading
Paragraph Comprehension
Passage Comprehension

Mathematics
Numbers and Operations
Algebraic Applications
Data Interpretation
Measurement
Metric Conversion

Science
Human Body Science
Life Science
Earth and Physical Science
Scientific Reasoning

English and Language Usage
English Grammar and Usage
Word meaning in Context
Spelling and Punctuation
Sentence Structure

While we seek to make our guide as comprehensive as possible, note that like all entrance exams, the HOBET® Exam might be adjusted at some future point. New material might be added, or content that is no longer relevant or applicable might be removed. It is always a good idea to give the materials you receive when you register to take the HOBET® a careful review.

It is also important to note that not all schools use all the modules or the same version. Make sure you know which version of the HOBET and which modules your school will be using so you do not waste valuable study time studying material that is no on your school's test!

The HOBET® Study Plan

Now that you have made the decision to take the HOBET, it is time to get started. Before you do another thing, you will need to figure out a plan of attack. The very best study tip is to start early! The longer the time period you devote to regular study practice, the more likely you will be to retain the material and be able to access it quickly. If you thought that 1x20 is the same as 2x10, guess what? It really is not, when it comes to study time. Reviewing material for just an hour per day over the course of 20 days is far better than studying for two hours a day for only 10 days. The more often you revisit a particular piece of information, the better you will know it. Not only will your grasp and understanding be better, but your ability to reach into your brain and quickly and efficiently pull out the tidbit you need, will be greatly enhanced as well.

The great Chinese scholar and philosopher Confucius believed that true knowledge could be defined as knowing both what you know and what you do not know. The first step in preparing for the HOBET® Exam is to assess your strengths and weaknesses. You may already have an idea of what you know and what you do not know, but evaluating yourself using our Self-Assessment modules for each of the three areas, math, english science and reading, will clarify the details.

Making a Study Schedule

In order to make your study time most productive you will need to develop a study plan. The purpose of the plan is to organize all the bits of pieces of information in such a way that you will not feel overwhelmed. Rome was not built in a day, and learning everything you will need to know to pass the HOBET® Exam is going to take time, too. Arranging the material you need to learn into manageable chunks is the best way to go. Each study session should make you feel as though you have succeeded in accomplishing your goal, and your goal is simply to learn what you planned to learn during that particular session. Try to organize the content in such a way that each study session builds on previous ones. That way, you will retain the information, be better able to access it, and review the previous bits and pieces at the same time.

Self-assessment

The Best Study Tip! The very best study tip is to start early! The longer you study regularly, the more you will retain and 'learn' the material. Studying for 1 hour per day for 20 days is far better than studying for 2 hours for 10 days.

What don't you know?

The first step is to assess your strengths and weaknesses.

You may already have an idea of where your weaknesses are, or you can take our Self-assessment modules for each of the areas, math, English, science and reading.

Below is a table to assess your exam readiness in each content area. You can fill this in now, and correct if necessary after completing the self-assessments, or fill it in after you have taken the self-assessments.

Exam Readiness Assessment

Exam Component	Rate 1 to 5
Reading	
Paragraph Comprehension	
Passage Comprehension	
English	
Grammar	
Word Meaning (Vocabulary - Meaning in Context)	
Spelling & Punctuation	
Sentence Structure	
Math	
Basic Math	
Algebra	
Data Interpretation	
Measurement	
Science	
Human Body Science (Anatomy and Physiology)	
Life Science (Biology, Ecology etc.)	
Earth and Physical Sciences	
Scientific Reasoning	

Making a Study Schedule

The key to making a study plan is to divide the material you need to learn into manageable size and learn it, while at the same time reviewing the material that you already know.

Using the table above, any scores of 3 or below, you need to spend time learning, going over and practicing this subject area. A score of 4 means you need to review the material, but you don't have to spend time re-learning. A score of 5 and you are OK with just an occasional review before the exam.

A score of 0 or 1 means you really need to work on this area and should allocate the most time and the highest priority. Some students prefer a 5-day plan and others a 10-day plan. It also depends on how much time you have until the exam.

Here is an example of a 5-day plan based on an example from the table above:

Basic Math: 1 Study 1 hour everyday – review on last day
Life Science: 3 Study 1 hour for 2 days then ½ hour a day, then review
Vocabulary: 4 Review every second day
Spelling: 2 Study 1 hour on the first day – then ½ hour everyday
Reading: 5 Review for ½ hour every other day
Algebra: 5 Review for ½ hour every other day
Human Body Science: 5 very confident – review a few times.

Using this example, here is a sample study plan which you can adapt to your own situation:

Day	Subject	Time
Monday		
Study	Basic Math	1 hour
Study	Spelling	1 hour
½ hour break		
Study	Life Sciences	1 hour
Review	Human Body Sciences	½ hour
Tuesday		
Study	Basic Math	1 hour
Study	Spelling	½ hour
½ hour break		
Study	Data Interpretation	½ hour
Review	Vocabulary	½ hour
Review	Grammar	½ hour
Wednesday		
Study	Basic Math	1 hour
Study	Spelling	½ hour
½ hour break		
Study	LIfe Sciences	½ hour
Review	Human Body Sciences	½ hour
Thursday		
Study	Basic Math	½ hour
Study	Spelling	½ hour
Review	Life Sciences	½ hour
½ hour break		
Review	Grammar	½ hour
Review	Vocabulary	½ hour
Friday		
Review	Basic Math	½ hour
Review	Spelling	½ hour
Review	Life Sciences	½ hour
½ hour break		
Review	Vocabulary	½ hour
Review	Grammar	½ hour

Practice Test Questions Set 1

Section I – Reading

Questions: 42
Time: 45 Minutes

Section II – Mathematics

Questions: 30
Time: 30 Minutes

Section III – English and Language Usage

Questions: 30
Time: 30 Minutes

Section IV –Science

Questions: 48
Time: 40 minutes

The questions below are not the same as you will find on the HOBET® - that would be too easy! And nobody knows what the questions will be and they change all the time. Below are general questions that cover the same subject areas as the HOBET®. So, while the format and exact wording of the questions may differ slightly, and change from year to year, if you can answer the questions below, you will have no problem with the HOBET®.

For the best results, take these practice test questions as if it were the real exam. Set aside time when you will not be disturbed, and a location that is quiet and free of distractions. Read the instructions carefully, read each question carefully, and answer to the best of your ability.

Use the bubble answer sheets provided. When you have completed the practice questions, check your answer against the Answer Key and read the explanation provided.

You are given 209 minutes to complete the full HOBET® exam.

Do not attempt more than one set of practice test questions in one day. After completing the first practice test, wait two or three days before attempting the second set of questions.

Section 1 - Reading

1. (A) (B) (C) (D)

2. (A) (B) (C) (D)

3. (A) (B) (C) (D)

4. (A) (B) (C) (D)

5. (A) (B) (C) (D)

6. (A) (B) (C) (D)

7. (A) (B) (C) (D)

8. (A) (B) (C) (D)

9. (A) (B) (C) (D)

10. (A) (B) (C) (D)

11. (A) (B) (C) (D)

12. (A) (B) (C) (D)

13. (A) (B) (C) (D)

14. (A) (B) (C) (D)

15. (A) (B) (C) (D)

16. (A) (B) (C) (D)

17. (A) (B) (C) (D)

18. (A) (B) (C) (D)

19. (A) (B) (C) (D)

20. (A) (B) (C) (D)

21. (A) (B) (C) (D)

22. (A) (B) (C) (D)

23. (A) (B) (C) (D)

24. (A) (B) (C) (D)

25. (A) (B) (C) (D)

26. (A) (B) (C) (D)

27. (A) (B) (C) (D)

28. (A) (B) (C) (D)

29. (A) (B) (C) (D)

30. (A) (B) (C) (D)

31. (A) (B) (C) (D)

32. (A) (B) (C) (D)

33. (A) (B) (C) (D)

34. (A) (B) (C) (D)

35. (A) (B) (C) (D)

36. (A) (B) (C) (D)

37. (A) (B) (C) (D)

38. (A) (B) (C) (D)

39. (A) (B) (C) (D)

40. (A) (B) (C) (D)

41. (A) (B) (C) (D)

42. (A) (B) (C) (D)

Section II - Math

1. (A) (B) (C) (D)   11. (A) (B) (C) (D)   21. (A) (B) (C) (D)

2. (A) (B) (C) (D)   12. (A) (B) (C) (D)   22. (A) (B) (C) (D)

3. (A) (B) (C) (D)   13. (A) (B) (C) (D)   23. (A) (B) (C) (D)

4. (A) (B) (C) (D)   14. (A) (B) (C) (D)   24. (A) (B) (C) (D)

5. (A) (B) (C) (D)   15. (A) (B) (C) (D)   25. (A) (B) (C) (D)

6. (A) (B) (C) (D)   16. (A) (B) (C) (D)   26. (A) (B) (C) (D)

7. (A) (B) (C) (D)   17. (A) (B) (C) (D)   27. (A) (B) (C) (D)

8. (A) (B) (C) (D)   18. (A) (B) (C) (D)   28. (A) (B) (C) (D)

9. (A) (B) (C) (D)   19. (A) (B) (C) (D)   29. (A) (B) (C) (D)

10. (A) (B) (C) (D)   20. (A) (B) (C) (D)   30. (A) (B) (C) (D)

Section III English

1. (A) (B) (C) (D)   11. (A) (B) (C) (D)   21. (A) (B) (C) (D)

2. (A) (B) (C) (D)   12. (A) (B) (C) (D)   22. (A) (B) (C) (D)

3. (A) (B) (C) (D)   13. (A) (B) (C) (D)   23. (A) (B) (C) (D)

4. (A) (B) (C) (D)   14. (A) (B) (C) (D)   24. (A) (B) (C) (D)

5. (A) (B) (C) (D)   15. (A) (B) (C) (D)   25. (A) (B) (C) (D)

6. (A) (B) (C) (D)   16. (A) (B) (C) (D)   26. (A) (B) (C) (D)

7. (A) (B) (C) (D)   17. (A) (B) (C) (D)   27. (A) (B) (C) (D)

8. (A) (B) (C) (D)   18. (A) (B) (C) (D)   28. (A) (B) (C) (D)

9. (A) (B) (C) (D)   19. (A) (B) (C) (D)   29. (A) (B) (C) (D)

10. (A) (B) (C) (D)   20. (A) (B) (C) (D)   30. (A) (B) (C) (D)

Section IV – Science

1. (A) (B) (C) (D)
2. (A) (B) (C) (D)
3. (A) (B) (C) (D)
4. (A) (B) (C) (D)
5. (A) (B) (C) (D)
6. (A) (B) (C) (D)
7. (A) (B) (C) (D)
8. (A) (B) (C) (D)
9. (A) (B) (C) (D)
10. (A) (B) (C) (D)
11. (A) (B) (C) (D)
12. (A) (B) (C) (D)
13. (A) (B) (C) (D)
14. (A) (B) (C) (D)
15. (A) (B) (C) (D)
16. (A) (B) (C) (D)
17. (A) (B) (C) (D)

18. (A) (B) (C) (D)
19. (A) (B) (C) (D)
20. (A) (B) (C) (D)
21. (A) (B) (C) (D)
22. (A) (B) (C) (D)
23. (A) (B) (C) (D)
24. (A) (B) (C) (D)
25. (A) (B) (C) (D)
26. (A) (B) (C) (D)
27. (A) (B) (C) (D)
28. (A) (B) (C) (D)
29. (A) (B) (C) (D)
30. (A) (B) (C) (D)
31. (A) (B) (C) (D)
32. (A) (B) (C) (D)
33. (A) (B) (C) (D)
34. (A) (B) (C) (D)

35. (A) (B) (C) (D)
36. (A) (B) (C) (D)
37. (A) (B) (C) (D)
38. (A) (B) (C) (D)
39. (A) (B) (C) (D)
40. (A) (B) (C) (D)
41. (A) (B) (C) (D)
42. (A) (B) (C) (D)
43. (A) (B) (C) (D)
44. (A) (B) (C) (D)
45. (A) (B) (C) (D)
46. (A) (B) (C) (D)
47. (A) (B) (C) (D)
48. (A) (B) (C) (D)
49. (A) (B) (C) (D)
50. (A) (B) (C) (D)

Questions 1 – 4 refer to the following passage.

Passage 1 - Infectious Disease

An infectious disease is a clinically evident illness resulting from the presence of pathogenic agents, such as viruses, bacteria, fungi, protozoa, multicellular parasites, and unusual proteins known as prions. Infectious pathologies are also called communicable diseases or transmissible diseases, due to their potential of transmission from one person or species to another by a replicating agent (as opposed to a toxin).

Transmission of an infectious disease can occur in many different ways. Physical contact, liquids, food, body fluids, contaminated objects, and airborne inhalation can all transmit infecting agents.

Transmissible diseases that occur through contact with an ill person, or objects touched by them, are especially infective, and are sometimes called contagious diseases. Communicable diseases that require a more specialized route of infection, such as through blood or needle transmission, or sexual transmission, are usually not regarded as contagious.

The term infectivity describes the ability of an organism to enter, survive and multiply in the host, while the infectiousness of a disease shows the comparative ease with which the disease is transmitted. An infection however, is not synonymous with an infectious disease, as an infection may not cause important clinical symptoms. [9]

1. What can we infer from the first paragraph in this passage?

    a. Sickness from a toxin can be easily transmitted from one person to another.

    b. Sickness from an infectious disease can be easily transmitted from one person to another.

    c. Few sicknesses are transmitted from one person to another.

    d. Infectious diseases are easily treated.

2. What are two other names for infections' pathologies?

a. Communicable diseases or transmissible diseases

b. Communicable diseases or terminal diseases

c. Transmissible diseases or preventable diseases

d. Communicative diseases or unstable diseases

3. What does infectivity describe?

a. The inability of an organism to multiply in the host.

b. The inability of an organism to reproduce.

c. The ability of an organism to enter, survive and multiply in the host.

d. The ability of an organism to reproduce in the host.

4. How do we know an infection is not synonymous with an infectious disease?

a. Because an infectious disease destroys infections with enough time.

b. Because an infection may not cause important clinical symptoms or impair host function.

c. We do not. The two are synonymous.

d. Because an infection is too fatal to be an infectious disease.

Questions 5 – 8 refer to the following passage.

Low Blood Sugar

As the name suggest, low blood sugar is low sugar levels in the bloodstream. This can occur when you have not eaten properly and undertake strenuous activity, or when you are very hungry. When Low blood sugar occurs regularly and is ongoing, it is a medical condition called hypoglycemia. This condition can occur in diabetics and in healthy adults.

Causes of low blood sugar can include excessive alcohol consumption, metabolic problems, stomach surgery, pancreas, liver or kidneys problems, as well as a side-effect of some medications.

Symptoms

There are different symptoms depending on the severity of the case.

Mild hypoglycemia can lead to feelings of nausea and hunger. The patient may also feel nervous, jittery and have fast heart beats. Sweaty skin, clammy and cold skin are likely symptoms.

Moderate hypoglycemia can result in a short tempered, confusion, nervousness, fear and blurring of vision. The patient may feel weak and unsteady.

Severe cases of hypoglycemia can lead to seizures, coma, fainting spells, nightmares, headaches, excessive sweats and severe tiredness.

Diagnosis of low blood sugar

A doctor can diagnosis this medical condition by asking the patient questions and testing blood and urine samples. Home testing kits are available for patients to monitor blood sugar levels. It is important to see a qualified doctor though. The doctor can administer tests to ensure that will safely rule out other medical conditions that could affect blood sugar levels.

Treatment

Quick treatments include drinking or eating foods and drinks with high sugar contents. Good examples include soda, fruit juice, hard candy and raisins. Glucose energy tablets can also help. Doctors may also recommend medications and well as changes in diet and exercise routine to treat chronic low blood sugar.

5. Based on the article, which of the following is true?

    a. Low blood sugar can happen to anyone.

    b. Low blood sugar only happens to diabetics.

    c. Low blood sugar can occur even.

    d. None of the statements are true.

6. Which of the following are the author's opinion?

    a. Quick treatments include drinking or eating foods and drinks with high sugar contents.

    b. None of the statements are opinions.

    c. This condition can occur in diabetics and in healthy adults.

    d. There are different symptoms depending on the severity of the case

7. What is the author's purpose?

    a. To inform

    b. To persuade

    c. To entertain

    d. To analyze

8. Which of the following is not a detail?

    a. A doctor can diagnosis this medical condition by asking the patient questions and testing.

    b. A doctor will test blood and urine samples.

    c. Glucose energy tablets can also help.

    d. Home test kits monitor blood sugar levels.

Questions 9 – 11 refer to the following passage.

Passage 3 – Thunderstorms

The first stage of a thunderstorm is the cumulus stage, or developing stage. In this stage, masses of moisture are lifted upwards into the atmosphere. The trigger for this lift can be insulation heating the ground producing thermals, areas where two winds converge, forcing air upwards, where winds blow over terrain of increasing elevation. Moisture in the air rapidly cools into liquid drops of water, which appears as cumulus clouds.

As the water vapor condenses into liquid, latent heat is released which warms the air, causing it to become less dense than the surrounding dry air. The warm air rises in an updraft through the process of convection (hence the term convective precipitation). This creates a low-pressure zone beneath the forming thunderstorm. In a typical thunderstorm, about 5×10^8 kg of water vapor is lifted, and the quantity of energy released when this condenses is about equal to the energy used by a city of 100,000 in a month. [10]

9. The cumulus stage of a thunderstorm is the

    a. The last stage of the storm.

    b. The middle stage of the storm formation.

    c. The beginning of the thunderstorm.

    d. The period after the thunderstorm has ended.

10. One of the ways the air is warmed is

    a. Air moving downwards, which creates a high-pressure zone.

    b. Air cooling and becoming less dense, causing it to rise.

    c. Moisture moving downward toward the earth.

    d. Heat created by water vapor condensing into liquid.

11. Identify the correct sequence of events

a. Warm air rises, water droplets condense, creating more heat, and the air rises further.

b. Warm air rises and cools, water droplets condense, causing low pressure.

c. Warm air rises and collects water vapor, the water vapor condenses as the air rises, which creates heat, and causes the air to rise farther.

d. None of the above.

Questions 12 – 14 refer to the following passage.

Passage 4 If You Have Allergies, You're Not Alone

People who experience allergies might joke that their immune systems have let them down or are seriously lacking. Truthfully though, people who experience allergic reactions or allergy symptoms during certain times of the year have heightened immune systems that are "better" than those of people who have perfectly healthy but less militant immune systems.

Still, when a person has an allergic reaction, they are having an adverse reaction to a substance that is considered normal to most people. Mild allergic reactions usually have symptoms like itching, runny nose, red eyes, or bumps or discoloration of the skin. More serious allergic reactions, such as those to animal and insect poisons or certain foods, may result in the closing of the throat, swelling of the eyes, low blood pressure, an inability to breathe, and can even be fatal.

Different treatments help different allergies, and which one a person uses depends on the nature and severity of the allergy. It is recommended to patients with severe allergies to take extra precautions, such as carrying an EpiPen, which treats anaphylactic shock and may prevent death, always in order for the remedy to be readily available and more effective. When an allergy is not so severe, treatments may be used just relieve a person of uncomfortable symptoms. Over the counter allergy medicines treat milder symptoms, and can be bought at any grocery store and used in moderation to help people with allergies live normally.

There are many tests available to assess whether a person has allergies or what they may be allergic to, and advances in these tests and the medicine used to treat patients continues to improve. Despite this fact, allergies still affect many people throughout the year or even every day. Medicines used to treat allergies have side effects of their own, and it is difficult to bring the body into balance with the use of medicine. Regardless, many of those who live with allergies are grateful for what is available and find it useful in maintaining their lifestyles.

12. According to this passage, it can be understood that the word "militant" belongs in a group with the words:

    a. sickly, ailing, faint

    b. strength, power, vigor

    c. active, fighting, warring

    d. worn, tired, breaking down

13. The author says that "medicines used to treat allergies have side effects of their own" in order to

    a. point out that doctors aren't very good at diagnosing and treating allergies

    b. argue that because of the large number of people with allergies, a cure will never be found

    c. explain these allergy medicines aren't cures, and some compromise must be made

    d. argue that more wholesome remedies should be researched and medicines banned

14. It can be inferred that _____ recommend that some people with allergies carry medicine with them.

    a. the author

    b. doctors

    c. the makers of EpiPen

    d. people with allergies

Questions 15 refers to the following Table of Contents.

Contents

15. Consider the table of contents above. What page would you find information about natural selection and adaptation?

    a. 81

    b. 90

    c. 110

    d. 132

Questions 16 – 19 refer to the following passage.

Passage 5 – Clouds

A cloud is a visible mass of droplets or frozen crystals floating in the atmosphere above the surface of the Earth or other
planetary bodies. Another type of cloud is a mass of material
in space, attracted by gravity, called interstellar clouds and
nebulae. The branch of meteorology which studies clouds is
called nephrology. When we are speaking of Earth clouds,
water vapor is usually the condensing substance, which
forms small droplets or ice crystal. These crystals are typi-
cally 0.01 mm in diameter. Dense, deep clouds reflect most
light, so they appear white, at least from the top. Cloud droplets scatter light very efficiently, so the farther into a cloud
light travels, the weaker it gets. This accounts for the gray
or dark appearance at the base of large clouds. Thin clouds
may appear to have acquired the color of their environment
or background. [11]

16. What are clouds made of?

    a. Water droplets

    b. Ice crystals

    c. Ice crystals and water droplets

    d. Clouds on Earth are made of ice crystals and water
droplets

17. The main idea of this passage is

    a. Condensation occurs in clouds, having an intense ef-
fect on the weather on the surface of the earth.

    b. Atmospheric gases are responsible for the gray color
of clouds just before a severe storm happens.

    c. A cloud is a visible mass of droplets or frozen crys-
tals floating in the atmosphere above the surface of the
Earth or other planetary body.

    d. Clouds reflect light in varying amounts and degrees,
depending on the size and concentration of the water
droplets.

18. The branch of meteorology that studies clouds is called

    a. Convection

    b. Thermal meteorology

    c. Nephology

    d. Nephelometry

19. Why are clouds white on top and grey on the bottom?

    a. Because water droplets inside the cloud do not reflect light, it appears white, and the farther into the cloud the light travels, the less light is reflected making the bottom appear dark.

    b. Because water droplets outside the cloud reflect light, it appears dark, and the farther into the cloud the light travels, the more light is reflected making the bottom appear white.

    c. Because water droplets inside the cloud reflects light, making it appear white, and the farther into the cloud the light travels, the more light is reflected making the bottom appear dark.

    d. None of the above.

Questions 20 - 23 refer to the following recipe.

"When a Poet Longs to Mourn, He Writes an Elegy"

Poems are an expressive, especially emotional, form of writing. They have been present in literature virtually from the time civilizations invented the written word. Poets often portrayed as moody, secluded, and even troubled, but this is because poets are introspective and feel deeply about the current events and cultural norms they are surrounded with. Poets often produce the most telling literature, giving insight into the society and mind-set they come from. This can be done in many forms.

The oldest types of poems often include many stanzas, may or may not rhyme, and are more about telling a story than experimenting with language or words. The most common types of ancient poetry are epics, which are usually extremely long stories that follow a hero through his journey, or ellegies, which are often solemn in tone and used to mourn or lament something or someone. The Mesopotamians are often said to have invented the written word, and their literature is among the oldest in the world, including the epic poem titled "Epic of Gilgamesh." Similar in style and length to "Gilgamesh" is "Beowulf," an ellegy poem written in Old English and set in Scandinavia. These poems are often used by professors as the earliest examples of literature.

The importance of poetry was revived in the Renaissance. At this time, Europeans discovered the style and beauty of ancient Greek arts, and poetry was among those. Shakespeare is the most well-known poet of the time, and he used poetry not only to write poems but also to write plays for the theater. The most popular forms of poetry during the Renaissance included villanelles, sonnets, as well as the epic. Poets during this time focused on style and form, and developed very specific rules and outlines for how an exceptional poem should be written.

As often happens in the arts, modern poets have rejected the constricting rules of Renaissance poets, and free form poems are much more popular. Some modern poems would read just like stories if they weren't arranged into lines and stanzas. It is difficult to tell which poems and poets will be the most important, because works of art often become more famous in hindsight, after the poet has died and society can look at itself without being in the moment. Modern poetry continues to develop, and will no doubt continue to change as values, thought, and writing continue to change.

Poems can be among the most enlightening and uplifting texts for a person to read if they are looking to connect with the past, connect with other people, or try to gain an understanding of what is happening in their time.

20. In summary, the author has written this passage

    a. as a foreword that will introduce a poem in a book or magazine

    b. because she loves poetry and wants more people to like it

    c. to give a brief history of poems

    d. to convince students to write poems

21. The author organizes the paragraphs mainly by

    a. moving chronologically, explaining which types of poetry were common in that time

    b. talking about new types of poems each paragraph and explaining them a little

    c. focusing on one poet or group of people and the poems they wrote

    d. explaining older types of poetry so she can talk about modern poetry

22. The author's claim that poetry has been around "virtually from the time civilizations invented the written word" is supported by the detail that

    a. Beowulf is written in Old English, which is not really in use any longer

    b. epic poems told stories about heroes

    c. the Renaissance poets tried to copy Greek poets

    d. the Mesopotamians are credited with both inventing the word and writing "Epic of Gilgamesh"

23. According to the passage, it can be understood that the word "telling" means

    a. speaking

    b. significant

    c. soothing

d. word**y**

Questions 24 – 25 refer to the following email.

SUBJECT: MEDICAL STAFF CHANGES

To all staff:

This email is to advise you of a paper on recommended medical staff changes has been posted to the Human Resources website.

The contents are of primary interest to medical staff, other staff may be interested in reading it, particularly those in medical support roles.

The paper deals with several major issues:

1. Improving our ability to attract top quality staff to the hospital, and retain our existing staff. These changes will make our position and departmental names internationally recognizable and comparable with North American and North Asian departments and positions.

2. Improving our ability to attract top quality staff by introducing greater flexibility in the departmental structure.

3. General comments on issues to be further discussed relative to research staff.

The changes outlined in this paper are significant. I encourage you to read the document and send to me any comments you may have, so that it can be enhanced and improved.

Gordon Simms
Administrator,
Seven Oaks Regional Hospital

24. Are all hospital staff required to read the document posted to the Human Resources website?

> a. Yes all staff are required to read the document.
>
> b. No, reading the document is optional.
>
> c. Only medical staff are required to read the document.
>
> d. None of the above are correct.

25. Have the changes to medical staff been made?

> a. Yes, the changes have been made.
>
> b. No, the changes are only being discussed.
>
> c. Some of the changes have been made.
>
> d. None of the choices are correct.

Questions 26 – 30 refer to the following passage.

Passage 8 – Navy Seals

The United States Navy's Sea, Air and Land Teams, commonly known as Navy SEALs, are the U.S. Navy's principal special operations force, and a part of the Naval Special Warfare Command (NSWC) as well as the maritime component of the United States Special Operations Command (USSOCOM).

The unit's acronym ("SEAL") comes from their capacity to operate at sea, in the air, and on land – but it is their ability to work underwater that separates SEALs from most other military units in the world. Navy SEALs are trained and have been deployed in a wide variety of missions, including direct action and special reconnaissance operations, unconventional warfare, foreign internal defence, hostage rescue, counter-terrorism and other missions. All SEALs are members of either the United States Navy or the United States Coast Guard.

In the early morning of May 2, 2011 local time, a team of 40

CIA-led Navy SEALs completed an operation to kill Osama bin Laden in Abbottabad, Pakistan about 35 miles (56 km) from Islamabad, the country's capital. The Navy SEALs were part of the Naval Special Warfare Development Group, previously called "Team 6." President Barack Obama later confirmed the death of bin Laden. The unprecedented media coverage raised the public profile of the SEAL community, particularly the counter-terrorism specialists commonly known as SEAL Team 6. [12]

26. Are Navy SEALs part of USSOCOM?

    a. Yes

    b. No

    c. Only for special operations

    d. No, they are part of the US Navy

27. What separates Navy SEALs from other military units?

    a. Belonging to NSWC

    b. Direct action and special reconnaissance operations

    c. Working underwater

    d. Working for other military units in the world

28. What other military organizations do SEALs belong to?

    a. The US Navy

    b. The Coast Guard

    c. The US Army

    d. The Navy and the Coast Guard

29. What other organization participated in the Bin Laden raid?

    a. The CIA

    b. The US Military

    c. Counter-terrorism specialists

    d. None of the above

30. What is the new name for Team 6?

    a. They were always called Team 6

    b. The counter-terrorism specialists

    c. The Naval Special Warfare Development Group

    d. None of the above

Questions 31 – 33 refer to the following passage.

Passage 9 - Gardening

Gardening for food extends far into prehistory. Ornamental gardens were known in ancient times, a famous example being the Hanging Gardens of Babylon, while ancient Rome had dozens of gardens.

The earliest forms of gardens emerged from the people's need to grow herbs and vegetables. It was only later that rich individuals created gardens for purely decorative purposes.

In ancient Egypt, rich people created ornamental gardens to relax in the shade of the trees. Egyptians believed that gods liked gardens. Commonly, walls surrounded ancient Egyptian gardens with trees planted in rows.
The most popular tree species were date palms, sycamores, fig trees, nut trees, and willows. Besides ornamental gardens, wealthy Egyptians kept vineyards to produce wine.

The Assyrians are also known for their beautiful gardens in what we know today as Iraq. Assyrian gardens were very large, with some of them used for hunting and others as leisure gardens. Cypress and palm were the most popular trees in Assyrian gardens. [13]

31. Why did wealthy people in Egypt have gardens?

    a. For food

    b. To relax in the shade

    c. For ornamentation

    d. For hunting

32. What did the Egyptians believe about gardens?

    a. They believed gods loved gardens.

    b. They believed gods hated gardens.

    c. The didn't have any beliefs about gods and Gardens.

    d. They believed gods hated trees.

33. What kinds of trees did the Assyrians like?

    a. The Assyrians liked date palms, sycamores, fig trees, nut trees, and willows.

    b. The Assyrians liked Cypresses and palms.

    c. The Assyrians didn't like trees.

    d. The Assyrians liked hedges and vines.

34. Which came first, gardening for vegetables or ornamental gardens?

    a. Ornamental gardens came before vegetable gardens.

    b. Vegetable gardens came before ornamental gardens.

    c. Vegetable and ornamental gardens appeared at the same time.

    d. The passage does not give enough information.

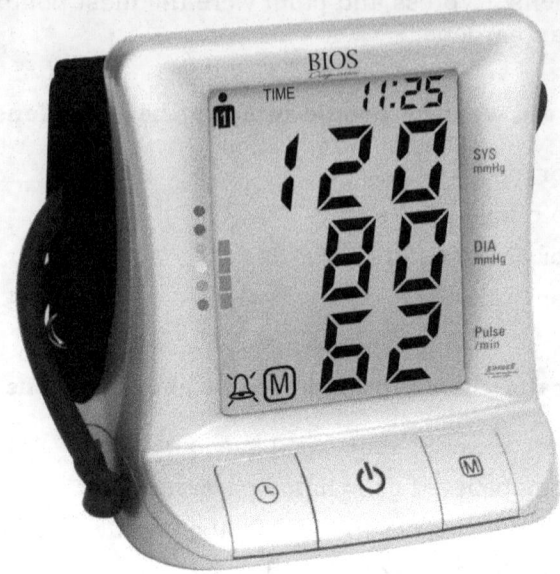

35. Consider the blood pressure gauge above. According to this gauge, what is the patient's pulse?

    a. 120 beats per minute

    b. 80 beats per minute

    c. 62 beats per minute

    d. The pulse is not shown

Questions 35 – 39 refer to the following passage.

Passage 10 - Gardens

Ancient Roman gardens are known for their statues and sculptures, which were never missing from the lives of Romans. Romans designed their gardens with hedges and vines as well as a wide variety of flowers, including acanthus, cornflowers and crocus, cyclamen, hyacinth, iris and ivy, lavender, lilies, myrtle, narcissus, poppy, rosemary and violet. Flower beds were popular in the courtyards of the rich

Romans.

The Middle Ages was a period of decline in gardening. After the fall of Rome, gardening was only for growing medicinal herbs and decorating church altars.

Islamic gardens were built after the model of Persian gardens, with enclosed walls and watercourses dividing the garden into four. Commonly, the center of the garden would have a pool or pavilion. Mosaics and glazed tiles used to decorate elaborate fountains are specific to Islamic gardens.
13

36. What is a characteristic feature of Roman gardens?

a. Statues and sculptures

b. Flower beds

c. Medicinal herbs

d. Courtyard gardens

37. When did gardening decline?

a. Before the Fall of Rome

b. Gardening did not decline

c. Before the Middle Ages

d. After the Fall of Rome

38. What kind of gardening was done during the Middle Ages?

a. Gardening with hedges and vines

b. Gardening with a wide variety of flowers

c. Gardening for herbs and church alters

d. Gardening divided by watercourses

39. What is a characteristic feature of Islamic Gardens?

    a. Statues and Sculptures

    b. Decorative tiles and fountains

    c. Herbs

    d. Flower beds

40. When folded, which shape is possible?

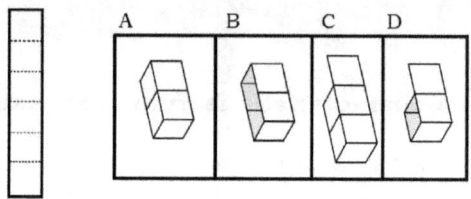

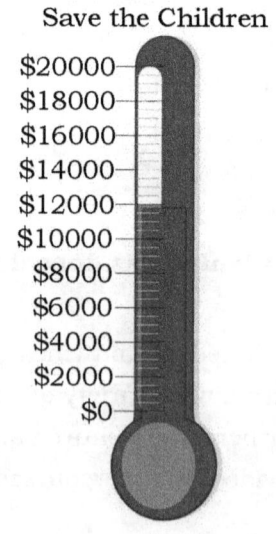

Save the Children

41. Consider the graphic above. The Save the Children fund has a fund-raising goal of $20,000. Approximately how much of their goal have they achieved?

    a. 3/5

    b. 3/4

    c. 1/2

    d. 1/3

42. Consider the graphic above. The Save the Children fund has a fund-raising goal of $16,000. About how much of their goal have they achieved?

    a. 3/5

    b. 3/4

    c. 1/2

    d. 1/3

Section II – Math

1. What is 1/3 of 3/4?

    a. 1/4

    b. 1/3

    c. 2/3

    d. 3/4

2. Susan wants to buy a leather jacket that costs $545.00 and is on sale for 10% off. What is the approximate cost?

    a. $525

    b. $450

    c. $475

    d. $500

3. 3.14 + 2.73 + 23.7 =

    a. 28.57

    b. 30.57

    c. 29.56

    d. 29.57

4. A woman spent 15% of her income on an item and ends with $120. What percentage of her income is left?

    a. 12%

    b. 85%

    c. 75%

    d. 95%

5. Express 0.27 + 0.33 as a fraction.

    a. 3/6

    b. 4/7

    c. 3/5

    d. 2/7

6. 8 is what percent of 40?

    a. 10%

    b. 15%

    c. 20%

    d. 25%

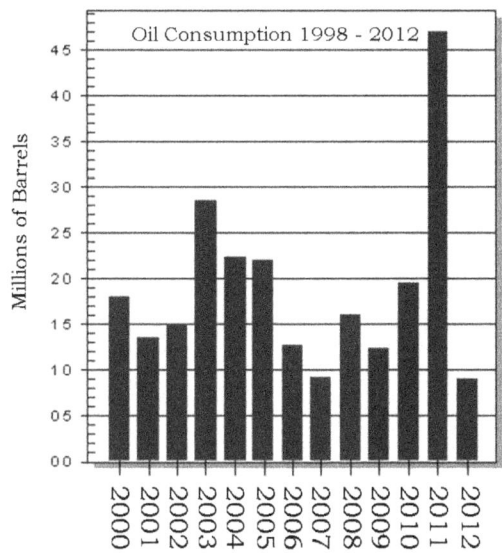

7. The graph above shows oil consumption in millions of barrels for the period, 1998 - 2012. What year did oil consumption peak?

    a. 2011

    b. 2010

    c. 2008

    d. 2009

8. Translate the following into an equation: 2 + a number divided by 7.

    a. $(2 + X)/7$

    b. $(7 + X)/2$

    c. $(2 + 7)/X$

    d. $2/(7 + X)$

Practice the HOBET®

9. .4% of 36 is

    a. 1.44

    b. .144

    c. 14.4

    d. 144

10. The physician ordered 5 mg Coumadin; 10 mg/tablet is on hand. How many tablets will you give?

    a. .5 tablet

    b. 1 tablet

    c. .75 tablet

    d. 1.5 tablets

11. The physician ordered 20 mg Tylenol/kg of body weight; on hand is 80 mg/tablet. The child weighs 12 kg. How many tablets will you give?

    a. 1 tablet

    b. 3 tablets

    c. 2 tablets

    d. 4 tablets

12. Consider the following population growth chart.

Country	Population 2000	Population 2005
Japan	122,251,000	128,057,000
China	1,145,195,000	1,341,335,000
United States	253,339,000	310,384,000
Indonesia	184,346,000	239,871,000

What country is growing the fastest?

    a. Japan

    b. China

    c. United States

    d. Indonesia

13. If y = 4 and x = 3, solve yx^3

    a. -108

    b. 108

    c. 27

    d. 4

14. What number is MCMXC?

    a. 1990

    b. 1980

    c. 2000

    d. 1995

15. Convert 16 quarts to gallons.

    a. 1 gallons

    b. 8 gallons

    c. 4 gallons

    d. 4.5 gallons

16. Convert 45 kg. to pounds.

    a. 10 pounds

    b. 100 pounds

    c. 1,000 pounds

    d. 110 pounds

17. Translate the following into an equation: three plus a number times 7 equals 42.

    a. $7(3 + X) = 42$

    b. $3(X + 7) = 42$

    c. $3X + 7 = 42$

    d. $(3 + 7)X = 42$

18. In a class of 83 students, 72 are present. What percent of the students are absent? Provide answer up to two significant digits.

    a. 12%

    b. 13%

    c. 14%

    d. 15%

19. $5x+2(x+7) = 14x - 7$. Find x

    a. 1

    b. 2

    c. 3

    d. 4

20. $5(z+1) = 3(z+2) + 11$. Find z

    a. 2

    b. 4

    c. 6

    d. 12

21. The price of a book went from $20 to $25. What percent did the price increase?

   a. 5%

   b. 10%

   c. 20%

   d. 25%

22. A boy is given 2 apples while his sister is given 8 oranges. What is the ratio between the boy's apples and her oranges?

   a. 1:2

   b. 2:4

   c. 1:4

   d. 2:1

23. In the time required to serve 43 customers, a server breaks 2 glasses and slips 5 times. The next day, the same server breaks 10 glasses. Assuming that glasses broken is proportional to customers served, how many customers did she serve?

   a. 25

   b. 43

   c. 86

   d. 215

24. A square lawn has an area of 62,500 square meters. What will the cost of building fence around it at a rate of $5.5 per meter?

   a. $4000

   b. $4500

   c. $5000

   d. $5500

25. Solve for n, when 5n + (19 − 2) = 67.

    a. 21

    b. 10

    c. 15

    d. 7

26. Below is the attendance for a class of 45.

Day	Absent Students
Monday	5
Tuesday	9
Wednesday	4
Thursday	10
Friday	6

What is the average attendance for the week?

    a. 88%

    b. 85%

    c. 81%

    d. 77%

27. A distributor purchased 550 kilograms of potatoes for $165. He distributed these at a rate of $6.4 per 20 kilograms to 15 shops, $3.4 per 10 kilograms to 12 shops and the remainder at $1.8 per 5 kilograms. If his total distribution cost is $10, what will his profit be?

    a. $10.40

    b. $8.60

    c. $14.90

    d. $23.40

28. How much pay does Mr. Johnson receive if he gives half of his pay to his family, $250 to his landlord, and has exactly 3/7 of his pay left over?

    a. $3600

    b. $3500

    c. $2800

    d. $1750

29. A boy has 4 red, 5 green and 2 yellow balls. He chooses two balls randomly. What is the probability that one is red and other is green?

    a. 2/11

    b. 19/22

    c. 20/121

    d. 9/11

30. The cost of waterproofing canvas is .50 a square yard. What's the total cost for waterproofing a canvas truck cover that is 15' x 24'?

    a. $18.00

    b. $6.67

    c. $180.00

    d. $20.00

Section III - English

1. Choose the sentence with the correct grammar.

a. Don would never have thought of that book, but you could have reminded him.

b. Don would never of thought of that book, but you could have reminded him.

c. Don would never have thought of that book, but you could of have reminded him.

d. Don would never of thought of that book, but you could of reminded him.

2. Choose the correct sentence.

a. The boy and girl are related.

b. The boy and girl is related.

c. The boy and girl was related.

d. None of the above.

3. Choose the sentence with the correct grammar.

a. There was scarcely no food in the pantry, because nobody ate at home.

b. There was scarcely any food in the pantry, because nobody ate at home.

c. There was scarcely any food in the pantry, because not nobody ate at home.

d. There was scarcely no food in the pantry, because not nobody ate at home.

4. Choose the sentence with the correct grammar.

a. Its important for you to know its official name; its called the Confederate Museum.

b. It's important for you to know it's official name; it's called the Confederate Museum.

c. It's important for you to know its official name; it's called the Confederate Museum.

d. Its important for you to know it's official name; it's called the Confederate Museum.

5. Choose the sentence with the correct grammar.

a. The man as well as his son has arrived.

b. The man as well as his son have arrived.

c. Both of the above.

d. None of the above.

6. Thomas Edison _____ since he invented the light bulb, television, motion pictures, and phonograph.

a. has always been known as the greatest inventor

b. was always been known as the greatest inventor

c. must have had been always known as the greatest inventor

d. will had been known as the greatest inventor

7. The weatherman on Channel 6 said that this has been the

a. most hottest summer on record

b. most hotter summer on record

c. hottest summer on record

d. hotter summer on record

8. Although Joe is tall for his age, his brother Elliot is _____ of the two.

    a. the tallest

    b. more tallest

    c. the tall

    d. the taller

9. When KISS came to town, all of the tickets _____ before I could buy one.

    a. will be sold out

    b. had been sold out

    c. were being sold out

    d. was sold out

10. The rules of most sports _____ more complicated than we often realize.

    a. are

    b. is

    c. was

    d. has been

11. _____ won first place in the Western Division?

    a. Who

    b. Whom

    c. Which

    d. What

12. There are now several ways to listen to music, including radio, CDs, and Mp3 files _____ you can download onto an MP3 player.

    a. on which

    b. who

    c. whom

    d. which

13. Choose the sentence with the correct grammar.

    a. Each of them have to be given a ticket.

    b. Each of them is to be given a ticket.

    c. Each of them are to be given a ticket.

    d. None of the above.

14. Choose the correct spelling.

    a. maintainance

    b. maintenace

    c. maintanance

    d. maintenance

15. Choose the correct spelling.

    a. humoros

    b. humouros

    c. humorous

    d. humorus

16. Choose the correct spelling.

    a. mathematics

    b. mathmatics

    c. matematics

    d. mathamatics

17. Choose the sentence below with the correct punctuation.

    a. Ted and Janice, who had been friends for years, went on vacation together every summer.

    b. Ted and Janice, who had been friends for years, went on vacation together, every summer.

    c. Ted, and Janice who had been friends for years, went on vacation together every summer.

    d. Ted and Janice who had been friends for years went on vacation together every summer.

18. Choose the sentence with the correct capitalization.

    a. The Sahara Desert is found in the northern part of Africa.

    b. The Sahara Desert is found in the Northern part of Africa.

    c. The Sahara desert is found in the northern part of Africa.

    d. The Sahara desert is found in the Northern part of Africa.

19. She went with him to the dance.

What is the subject of this sentence?

    a. She

    b. Dance

    c. Him

    d. With

20. She studied long and hard and her marks showed it.

What is the predicate of this sentence?

    a. Studied long and hard

    b. Marks showed it

    c. Showed it

    d. None of the above

21. What is on the test?

What type of sentence is this?

    a. Imperative

    b. Interrogative

    c. Exclamatory

    d. Declarative

22. The aquarium featured brightly-colored tropical fish that came from the tropics.

What part of this sentence is redundant?

    a. Brightly-colored

    b. Tropical fish

    c. That came from the tropics

    d. Aquarium

23. Choose the correct sentence.

    a. Historians have been guessing the doctor was a woman for more than 100 years.

    b. Historians have been guessing for more than 100 years the doctor was a woman.

    c. Historians guessed the doctor was a woman for more than 100 years.

    d. None of the above.

24. Choose the correct sentence.

a. None of us want to go to the party not even, if there will be live music.

b. None of us want to go to the party, not even if there will be live music.

c. None of us want to go to the party not even if there will be live music.

d. None of us want to go to the party; not even if there will be live music.

25. Choose the correct sentence.

a. I own two dogs, a cat named Jeffrey, and Henry, the goldfish.

b. I own two dogs a cat, named Jeffrey, and Henry, the goldfish.

c. I own two dogs, a cat named Jeffrey; and Henry, the goldfish.

d. I own two dogs, a cat, named Jeffrey and Henry, the goldfish.

26. Choose the correct sentence.

a. During the years he was President, the country fought two wars.

b. During the years he was president, the country fought two wars.

c. During the years he was president, the Country fought two wars.

d. During the years he was President, the Country fought two wars.

27. Alice <u>jumped</u> when she saw the rabbit.

What part of speech is the underlined word?

    a. Noun

    b. Verb

    c. Adjective

    d. Adverb

28. Which of the following sentences contains a redundant phrase?

    a. I will be leaving shortly.

    b. I think the situation calls for a direct confrontation.

    c. The fish swam upstream with great difficulty.

    d. None of the above.

Directions: For each of the questions below, choose the word with the meaning best suited to the sentence based on the context.

29. Paul's rose bushes were being destroyed by Japanese beetles, so he invested in a good _____.

    a. Fungicide

    b. Fertilizer

    c. Sprinkler

    d. Pesticide

30. Because of a pituitary dysfunction, Karl lacked the necessary _____ to grow as tall as his father.

    a. Glands

    b. Hormones

    c. Vitamins

    d. Testosterone

Section III – Science

1. Describe the differences between genotypes and phenotypes.

    a. Phenotype refers to observed properties of an organism and genotype refers to the genes of an organism.

    b. Genotype refers to observed properties of an organism and phenotype refers to the genes of an organism.

    c. Phenotype refers to the DNA of an organism and genotype refers to the genes of an organism.

    d. Genotype refers to the DNA of an organism and phenotype refers to the genes of an organism.

2. A solution with a pH value of greater than 7 is

    a. Base.

    b. Acid.

    c. Neutral.

    d. None of the above.

3. Which statement below regarding Eukaryotic and prokaryotic cells is correct?

    a. Both are organelles

    b. Eukaryotic are not organelles

    c. Both have DNA

    d. Both have single membrane compartments

4. When we say that important traits for scientific classification are homologous, "homologous" means

a. Being shared among two or more animals with the same parent.

b. Being coincidentally shared by two totally different creatures.

c. Being inherited by the organisms' common ancestors.

d. Mutating beyond all reasonable expectations.

5. The manner in which instructions for building proteins, the basic structural molecules of living material are written in the DNA, is

a. Genotypic assignment.

b. Chromosome pattern.

c. Genetic code.

d. Genetic fingerprinting.

6. A _____ is a unit of inherited material, encoded by a strand of DNA and transcribed by RNA.

a. Allele

b. Phenotype

c. Gene

d. Genotype

7. Which, if any, of the following statements about meiosis are correct?

a. During meiosis, the number of chromosomes in the cell are halved.

b. Meiosis only occurs in eukaryotic cells.

c. Meiosis is the part of the life cycle that involves sexual reproduction.

d. All of these statements are correct.

8. A population of wolves expanded exponentially after a hunting ban. Within a few generations, their habitat exceeded its _____ _____.

    a. Carrying capacity

    b. Food source

    c. Population limit

    d. Supply capability

9. When a pouch in the large intestine becomes inflamed, this becomes an affliction known as

    a. Diverticulosis.

    b. Diverticulitis.

    c. Acid Reflux.

    d. Colon Cancer.

10. Why is detection of pathogens complicated?

    a. They evolve so quickly

    b. They die so quickly

    c. They are invisible

    d. They multiply so quickly

11. Photosynthesis is

    a. The process by which plants generate oxygen from carbon dioxide.

    b. The process by which plants generate carbon dioxide from oxygen.

    c. The process by which plants generate carbon dioxide and oxygen.

    d. None of the above.

12. Which, if any, of the following statements are false?

a. A mutation is a permanent change in the DNA sequence of a gene.

b. Mutations in a gene's DNA sequence can alter the amino acid sequence of the protein encoded by the gene.

c. Mutations in DNA sequences usually occur spontaneously.

d. Mutations in DNA sequences is caused by exposure to environmental agents such as sunshine.

13. Starting with the weakest, arrange the fundamental forces of nature in order of strength.

a. Gravity, Weak Nuclear Force, Electromagnetic Force, Strong Nuclear Force

b. Weak Nuclear Force, Gravity, Electromagnetic Force, Strong Nuclear Force

c. Strong Nuclear Force, Weak Nuclear Force, Electromagnetic Force, Gravity

d. Gravity, Strong Nuclear Force, Weak Nuclear Force, Electromagnetic Force

14. _____, which refers to the repeatability of measurement, does not require knowledge of the correct or true value.

a. Precision

b. Value

c. Certainty

d. Accuracy

15. Artificial selection

a. Is a process where desirable traits are systematically bred.

b. Is a process where traits become more or less common in a population.

c. Is a process where behaviors are favored.

d. None of the above.

16. Which of the following are not examples of vaporization?

a. Boiling

b. Evaporation

c. Condensation

d. All of the above

17. Describe the periodic table.

a. The periodic table is a tabular display of the chemical compounds organized on the basis of their atomic numbers, electron configurations, and recurring chemical properties.

b. The periodic table is a tabular display of the chemical elements, organized on the basis of their atomic numbers, electron configurations, and recurring chemical properties.

c. The periodic table is a tabular display of the chemical subatomic particles, organized on the basis of their atomic numbers, electron configurations, and recurring chemical properties.

d. None of the above.

**18. In terms of the scientific method, the term
_____ refers to the act of noticing or perceiving
something and/or recording a fact or occurrence.**

    a. Observation

    b. Diligence

    c. Perception

    d. Control

19. What is the difference, of any, between kinetic energy and potential energy?

    a. Kinetic energy is the energy of a body resulting from heat while potential energy is the energy possessed by an object that is chilled.

    b. Kinetic energy is the energy of a body resulting from motion while potential energy is the energy possessed by an object by virtue of its position or state, e.g., as in a compressed spring.

    c. There is no difference between kinetic and potential energy; all energy is the same.

    d. Potential energy is the energy of a body resulting from motion while kinetic energy is the energy possessed by an object by virtue of its position or state, e.g., as in a compressed spring.

20. What is the sequence of developmental stages through which members of a given species must pass?

    a. Life cycle

    b. Life expectancy

    c. Life sequence

    d. None of the above

21. Which one of the following best describes the function of a cell membrane?

a. It controls the substances entering and leaving the cell.

b. It keeps the cell in shape.

c. It controls the substances entering the cell.

d. It supports the cell structures.

22. Which of these is not a rank within the area of classification or taxonomy?

a. Species

b. Family

c. Genus

d. Relative position

23. A _____ is a statistic used as a measure of the dispersion or variation in a distribution.

a. Normal distribution

b. Range

c. Outlier

d. Standard deviation

24. Substances that deactivate catalysts are called

a. Inhibitors.

b. Catalytic poisons.

c. Positive catalysts.

d. None of the above.

25. Describe kinetic energy.

a. Kinetic energy is the energy an object possesses due to its mass.

b. Kinetic energy is the energy an object possesses due to its motion.

c. Kinetic energy is the energy an object possesses due to its chemical properties.

d. Kinetic energy is the stored energy an object possesses.

26. The interval of confidence around the measured value, such that the measured value is certain not to lie outside this stated interval, refers to the _____ of that value.

a. Accuracy

b. Error

c. Uncertainty

d. Measurement

27. What are the differences, if any, between arteries, veins, and capillaries?

a. Veins carry oxygenated blood away from the heart, arteries return oxygen-depleted blood to the heart, and capillaries are thin-walled blood vessels in which gas/ nutrient/ waste exchange occurs.

b. Capillaries carry oxygenated blood away from the heart, veins return oxygen-depleted blood to the heart, and capillaries are thin-walled blood vessels in which gas/ nutrient/ waste exchange occurs.

c. There are no differences; all perform the same function in different parts of the body.

d. Arteries carry oxygenated blood away from the heart, veins return oxygen-depleted blood to the heart, and capillaries are thin-walled blood vessels in which gas/ nutrient/ waste exchange occurs.

28. What part of the body starts inhalation?

    a. The lungs

    b. The diaphragm

    c. The larynx

    d. The kidneys

29. Another term for biological classification is:

    a. Darwinian classification.

    b. Animal classification.

    c. Molecular classification.

    d. Scientific classification.

30. What type of gene is not expressed as a trait unless inherited by both parents?

    a. Principal gene

    b. Latent gene

    c. Recessive gene

    d. Dominant gene

31. A _____ _____ is an approximation or simulation of a real system that omits all but the most essential variables of the system.

    a. Scientific method

    b. Independent variable

    c. Control group

    d. Scientific model

32. Neutrons are necessary within an atomic nucleus because

    a. They bind with protons via nuclear force.

    b. They bind with nuclei via nuclear force.

    c. They bind with protons via electromagnetic force.

    d. They bind with nuclei via electromagnetic force.

33. Which of the following statements is false?

    a. Most enzymes are proteins

    b. Enzymes are catalysts

    c. Most enzymes are inorganic

    d. Enzymes are large biological molecules

34. _____ are compounds that contain hydrogen, can dissolve in water to release hydrogen ions into solution, and, in an aqueous solution, can conduct electricity.

    a. Caustics

    b. Bases

    c. Acids

    d. Salts

35. What are the basic structural units of nucleic acids (DNA or RNA) whose sequence determines individual hereditary characteristics?

    a. Gene

    b. Nucleotide

    c. Phosphate

    d. Nitrogen base

36. List the classifications of organisms in order of size.

a. Genus, Kingdom, Phylum/division, Class, Order, and Family Species

b. Order, Kingdom, Phylum/division, Genus, Class, and Family Species

c. Genus, Kingdom, Phylum/division, Class, Order, and Family Species

d. Kingdom ,Genus, Phylum/division, Class, Order, and Family Species

e. Family species, Order, Class, Phylum/division, Kingdom, and Genus

37. Where does digestion begin?

a. In the throat

b. In the stomach

c. In the intestines

d. In the mouth

38. What are the main components of the circulatory system?

a. The heart, veins and blood vessels

b. The heart, brain, and ears

c. The nose, throat and ears

d. The lungs, stomach, and kidneys

39. What is an example of a pathogen that the immune system detects?

a. An atom

b. A molecule

c. A vitamin

d. A virus

40. Explain chemical bonds.

a. Chemical bonds are attractions between atoms that form chemical substances containing two or more atoms.

b. Chemical bonds are attractions between protons that form chemical elements containing two or more atoms.

c. Chemical bonds are two or more atoms that form chemical substances.

d. None of the above.

41. Which of these is not an example of a function of the stomach in digestion?

a. Storing food

b. Cleansing food of impurities

c. Mixing food with digestive juices

d. Transferring food into the intestines

42. The exchange of oxygen for carbon dioxide takes place in the alveolar area of

a. The throat.

b. The ears.

c. The appendix.

d. The lungs.

43. The number of protons in the nucleus of an atom is the

a. Atomic mass.

b. Atomic weight.

c. Atomic number.

d. None of the above.

44. Natural selection is

a. A process where biological traits become more common in a population.

b. A process where biological traits become less common in a population.

c. A process where biological traits become more or less common in a population.

d. None of the above.

45. Sex chromosomes are designated as being "X" or "Y" chromosomes. In terms of sex chromosomes, what differences exist between males and females?

a. Females have two X chromosomes and males have one X chromosome and one Y chromosome.

b. Females have one X chromosome, and males have one X chromosome and one Y chromosome.

c. Females have one Y chromosome, while males have one X chromosome.

d. Females have one X chromosome and one Y chromosome, and males have two X chromosomes.

46. How does the immune system fight off disease?

a. By identifying and killing tumor cells and pathogens.

b. By creating new blood cells that fight disease.

c. By expelling infection through the blood stream.

d. By giving you energy to resist disease infections.

47. Identify the chemical properties of water.

a. Water has two hydrogen atoms covalently bonded to one oxygen atom.

b. Water has two oxygen atoms covalently bonded to one hydrogen atom.

c. Water has two hydrogen atoms polar covalently bonded to one oxygen atom.

d. Water has two oxygen atoms polar covalently bonded to one hydrogen atom.

48. Which of the following is not true of atomic theory?

a. Originated in the early 19th century with the work of John Dalton.

b. Is the field of physics that describes the characteristics and properties of atoms that make up matter.

c. Explains temperature as the momentum of atoms.

d. Explains macroscopic phenomena through the behavior of microscopic atoms.

Practice Test 1 - Quick Reference Answer Key

Section 1 – Reading

1. B
2. A
3. C
4. B
5. A
6. B
7. A
8. A
9. C
10. D
11. A
12. C
13. C
14. B
15. C
16. D
17. C
18. C
19. C
20. C
21. A
22. D
23. B
24. B
25. B
26. A
27. C
28. D
29. A
30. C
31. B
32. A
33. B
34. B

35. C
36. A
37. D
38. C
39. B
40. B
41. A
42. B

Section II – Math

1. A
2. D
3. D
4. B
5. C
6. C
7. A
8. A
9. B
10. A
11. B
12. D
13. B
14. A
15. C
16. B
17. A
18. B
19. C
20. C
21. D
22. C
23. D
24. D
25. B
26. B
27. B
28. B
29. A
30. D

Section III English

1. A
2. A
3. B
4. C
5. A
6. A
7. C
8. D
9. B
10. A
11. A
12. D
13. B
14. D
15. C
16. A
17. A
18. A
19. A
20. A
21. B
22. C
23. B
24. B
25. A
26. B
27. B
28. B
29. D
30. B

Section IV – Science

1. A
2. A
3. A
4. C
5. C

6. C
7. D
8. A
9. B
10. A
11. A
12. C
13. A
14. A
15. A
16. C
17. B
18. A
19. B
20. A
21. A
22. D
23. D
24. B
25. B
26. C
27. D
28. B
29. D
30. C
31. D
32. A
33. C
34. C
35. A
36. A
37. D
38. A
39. D
40. A
41. B
42. D
43. C
44. C
45. A
46. A
47. A
48. C

Answer Key with Explanations

Section 1 – Reading

1. B
We can infer from this passage that sickness from an infectious disease can be easily transmitted from one person to another.

From the passage, "Infectious pathologies are also called communicable diseases or transmissible diseases, due to their potential of transmission from one person or species to another by a replicating agent (as opposed to a toxin)."

2. A
Two other names for infectious pathologies are communicable diseases and transmissible diseases.

From the passage, "Infectious pathologies are also called communicable diseases or transmissible diseases, due to their potential of transmission from one person or species to another by a replicating agent (as opposed to a toxin)."

3. C
Infectivity describes the ability of an organism to enter, survive and multiply in the host. This is taken directly from the passage, and is a definition type question.

Definition type questions can be answered quickly and easily by scanning the passage for the word you are asked to define.

"Infectivity" is an unusual word, so it is quick and easy to scan the passage looking for this word.

4. B
We know an infection is not synonymous with an infectious disease because an infection may not cause important clinical symptoms or impair host function.

5. A
Low blood sugar occurs both in diabetics and healthy adults.

6. B
None of the statements are the author's opinion.

7. A
The author's purpose is to inform.

8. A
The only statement that is **not** a detail is, "A doctor can diagnosis this medical condition by asking the patient questions and testing."

9. C
The cumulus stage of a thunderstorm is the beginning of the thunderstorm.

This is taken directly from the passage, "The first stage of a thunderstorm is the cumulus, or developing stage."

10. D
The passage lists four ways that air is heated. One way is, heat created by water vapor condensing into liquid.

11. A
The sequence of events can be taken from these sentences:

As the moisture carried by the [1] air currents rises, it rapidly cools into liquid drops of water, which appear as cumulus clouds. As the water vapor condenses into liquid, it [2] releases heat, which warms the air. This in turn causes the air to become less dense than the surrounding dry air and [3] rise farther.

12. C
This question tests the reader's vocabulary skills. The uses of the negatives "but" and "less," especially right next to each other, may confuse readers into answering with choices A or D, which list words that are the opposite of "militant." Readers may also be confused by the comparison of healthy people with what is being described as an overly healthy person -- both people are good, but the reader may look for which one is "worse" in the comparison, and therefore stray

toward the opposite words.

One key to understanding the meaning of "militant" is to look at the root; and then easily associate it with "military" and gain a sense of what the word signifies: defense (especially considered that the immune system defends the body). Choice C is correct over B because "militant" is an adjective, just as the words in C are, whereas the words in choice B are nouns.

13. C
This question tests the reader's understanding of function within writing. The other choices are details included in the surrounding the quoted text, and may therefore confuse the reader. Choice A somewhat contradicts what is said earlier in the paragraph, which is, that tests and treatments are improving, and probably doctors are along with them, but the paragraph doesn't actually mention doctors, and the subject of the question is the medicine. Choice B may seem correct to readers who aren't careful to understand that, while the author does mention the large number of people affected, the author is touching on the realities of living with allergies rather than about the likelihood of curing all allergies. Similarly, while the author does mention the "balance" of the body, which is easily associated with "wholesome," the author is not really making an argument and especially is not making an extreme statement that allergy medicines should be outlawed. Again, because the article's tone is on living with allergies, choice C is an appropriate choice that fits with the title and content of the text.

14. B
This question tests the reader's inference skills. The text does not state who is doing the recommending, but the use of the "patients," as well as the general context of the passage, lends itself to the logical partner, "doctors," choice B.

The author does mention the recommendation but doesn't present it as her own (i.e. "I recommend that"), so choice A may be eliminated. It may seem plausible that people with allergies (choice D) may recommend medicines or products to other people with allergies, but the text does not necessarily support this interaction taking place. Choice C may be selected because the EpiPen is specifically mentioned, but the use of the phrase "such as" when it is introduced is not limiting enough to assume the recommendation is coming from its creators.

15. C
You would find information about natural selection and adaptation in the ecology section which begins on page 110.

16. D
Clouds on Earth are made of water droplets or ice crystals. Clouds in space are made of different materials attracted by gravity.

Choice D is the best answer. Notice also that Choice D is the most specific.

17. C
The main idea is the first sentence of the passage; a cloud is a visible mass of droplets or frozen crystals floating in the atmosphere above the surface of the Earth or other planetary body.

The main idea is very often the first sentence of the paragraph.

18. C
Nephology, which is the study of cloud physics.

19. C
This question asks about the process, and gives choices that can be confirmed or eliminated easily.

From the passage, "Dense, deep clouds reflect most light, so they appear white, at least from the top. Cloud droplets scatter light very efficiently, so the farther into a cloud light travels, the weaker it gets. This accounts for the gray or dark appearance at the base of large clouds."

We can eliminate choice A, since water droplets inside the cloud do not reflect light is false.

We can eliminate choice B, since, water droplets outside the cloud reflect light, it appears dark, is false.

20. C

This question tests the reader's summarizing skills. The use of the word "actually" in describing what kind of people poets are, as well as other moments like this, may lead readers to selecting choices B or D, but the author is giving more information than trying to persuade readers. The author gives no indication that she loves poetry (B) or that people, students specifically (D), should write poems. Choice A is incorrect because the style and content of this paragraph do not match those of a foreword; forewords usually focus on the history or ideas of a specific poem to introduce it more fully and help it stand out against other poems. The author here focuses on several poems and gives broad statements. Instead, she tells a kind of story about poems, giving three very broad time periods in which to discuss them, thereby giving a brief history of poetry, as choice C states.

21. A

This question tests the reader's summarizing skills. Key words in the topic sentences of each of the paragraphs ("oldest," "Renaissance," "modern") should give the reader an idea that the author is moving chronologically. The opening and closing sentence-paragraphs are broad and talk generally. Choice B seems reasonable, but epic poems are mentioned in two paragraphs, eliminating the idea that only new types of poems are used in each paragraph. Choice C is also easily eliminated because the author clearly mentions several different poets, groups of people, and poems. Choice D also seems reasonable, considering that the author does move from older forms of poetry to newer forms, but use of "so (that)" makes this statement false, for the author gives no indication that she is rushing (the paragraphs are about the same size) or that she prefers modern poetry.

22. D

This question tests the reader's attention to detail. The key word is "invented"--it ties together the Mesopotamians, who invented the written word, and the fact that they, as the inventors, also invented and used poetry. The other selections focus on other details mentioned in the passage, such as that the Renaissance's admiration of the Greeks (C) and that Beowulf is in Old English (A). Choice B may seem like an attractive answer because it is unlike the others and because the idea of heroes seems rooted in ancient and early civilizations.

23. B
This question tests the reader's vocabulary and contextual-ization skills. "Telling" is not an unusual word, but it may be used here in a way that is not familiar to readers, as an adjective rather than a verb in gerund form. Choice A may seem like the obvious answer to a reader looking for a verb to match the use they are familiar with. If the reader under-stands that the word is being used as an adjective and that A is a ploy, they may opt to select choice D, "wordy," but it does not make sense in context. Choice C can be easily elim-inated, and doesn't have any connection to the paragraph or passage. "Significant" (B) does make sense contextually, especially relative to the phrase "give insight" used later in the sentence.

24. B
Reading the document posted to the Human Resources web-site is optional.

25. B
The document is recommended changes and have not be implemented yet.

26. A
Navy SEALs are the maritime component of the United States Special Operations Command (USSOCOM).

27. C
Working underwater separates SEALs from other military units. This is taken directly from the passage.

28. D
SEALs also belong to the Navy and the Coast Guard.

29. A
The CIA also participated. From the passage, the raid was conducted by a "team of 40 *CIA-led* Navy SEALS."

30. C
From the passage, "The Navy SEALs were part of the Naval Special Warfare Development Group, previously called 'Team 6.' "

31. B
This question is taken directly from the passage. Scan the passage for the word "Egypt" to find the answer quickly.

32. A
The Egyptians believed gods loved gardens.

33. B
Cypresses and palms were the most popular trees in Assyrian Gardens.

34. B
Vegetable gardens came before ornamental gardens.

The earliest forms of gardens emerged from the people's need to grow herbs and vegetables. It was only later that rich individuals created gardens for the purely decorative purpose.

35. C
According to the blood pressure gauge, the patient's pulse is 62 beats per minute.

36. A
The ancient Roman gardens are known for their statues and sculptures ... from the first sentence.

37. D
After the fall of Rome, gardening was only for medicinal purposes, AND gardening declined in the Middle Ages, so we can infer gardening declined after the fall of Rome.

38. C
From the passage, "After the fall of Rome gardening was only done with the purpose of growing medicinal herbs and decorating church altars," so Choice C.

39. B
From the passage, "Mosaics and glazed tiles used to decorate elaborate fountains are specific to Islamic gardens."

40. B
When folded the given form will result in choice B.

41. A
The Save the Children's fund has raised $12,000 out of
$20,000, or 12/20. Simplifying, 12/20 = 3/5

42. B
The Save the Children's fund has raised $12,000 out of
$16,000, or 12/16. Simplifying, 12/16 = 3/4.

Section II – Math

1. A
1/3 X 3/4 = 3/12 = 1/4
To multiply fractions, multiply the numerator and denominator.

2. D
The question asks for approximate cost, so work with round
numbers. The jacket costs $545.00 so we can round up
to $550. 10% of $550 is 55. We can round down to $50,
which is easier to work with. $550 - $50 is $500. The
jacket will cost about $500.

The actual cost will be 10% X 545 = $54.50
545 – 54.50 = $490.50

3. D
3.14 + 2.73 = 5.87 and 5.87 + 23.7 = 29.57

4. B
Spent 15%, so 100% - 15% = 85%

5. C
To convert a decimal to a fraction, take the places of decimal
as your denominator, here, 2, so in 0.27, '7' is in the 100th
place, so the fraction is 27/100 and 0.33 becomes 33/100.

Next estimate the answer quickly to eliminate obvious wrong
choices. 27/100 is about 1/4 and 33/100 is 1/3. 1/3 is
slightly larger than 1/4, and 1/4 + 1/4 is 1/2, so the answer

will be slightly larger than 1/2.
Looking at the choices, Choice A can be eliminated since 3/6
= 1/2. Choice D, 2/7 is less than 1/2 and be eliminated.
The answer is going to be Choice B or Choice C.

Do the calculation, 0.27 + 0.33 = 0.60 and 0.60 = 60/100 =
3/5, Choice C is correct.

6. C

This is an easy question, and shows how you can solve some
questions without doing the calculations. The question is, 8
is what percent of 40. Take easy percentages for an approximate answer and see what you get.

10% is easy to calculate because you can drop the zero, or
move the decimal point. 10% of 40 = 4, and 8 = 2 X 4, so, 8
must be 2 X 10% = 20%.

Here are the calculations which confirm the quick approximation.
8/40 = X/100 = 8 * 100 / 40X = 800/40 = X = 20

7. A

According to the graph, oil consumption peaked in 2011.

8. A

2 + a number divided by 7.
(2 + X) divided by 7.
(2 + X)/7

9. B

.4/100 * 36 = .4 * 36/100 = .144

10. A

5 mg/10/mg X 1 tab/1 = .5 tablets

11. B

Step 1: Set up the formula to calculate the dose to be given
in mg as per weight of the child:- Dose ordered X Weight in
Kg = Dose to be given
Step 2: 20 mg X 12 kg = 240 mg
240 mg/80 mg X 1 tab/1 = 240/80 = 3 tablets

12. D
Indonesia is growing the fastest at about 30%.

13. B
$(4)(3)^3 = (4)(27) = 108$

14. A
MCMXC is 1990. $1000 + (1000 - 100) + (100 - 10) = 1990$

15. C
4 quarts = 1 gallon, 16 quarts = 16/4 = 4 gallons. Conversion problems are easy to get confused. One way to think of them is which is larger - quarts or gallons? Gallons are larger, so if you are converting from quarts to gallons the number of gallons will be a smaller number. Keeping that in mind, you can do a 'common-sense' check your answer.

16. B
0.45 kg = 1 pound, 1 kg. = 1/0.45 and 45 kg = 1/0.45 x 45 = 99.208, or 100 pounds.

17. A
Three plus a number times 7 equals 42. Let X be the number.
(3 + X) times 7 = 42
7(3 + X) = 42

18. B
Number of absent students = 83 – 72 = 11

Percentage of absent students is found by proportioning the number of absent students to total number of students in the class = 11•100/83 = 13.25

Checking the answers, we round 13.25 to the nearest whole number: 13%

19. C
To solve for x, first simplify the equation
5x + 2x + 14 = 14x – 7
7x - 14x = -14 -7
-7x = -21
x = -21/-7
x = 3

20. C
$5z + 5 = 3z + 6 + 11$
$5z -3z + 5 = 6 + 11$
$5z - 3z = 6 + 11 -5$
$2z = 17 - 5$
$2z = 12$
$z = 12/2$
$z = 6$

21. D
Price increased by $5 ($25-$20). To calculate the percent increase:
$5/20 = X/100$
$500 = 20X$
$X = 500/20$
$X = 25\%$

22. C
The ratio is 2 to 8, or 1:4.

23. D
2 glasses are broken for 43 customers so 1 glass breaks for every $43/2$ customers served, therefore 10 glasses implies $(43/2)•10 = 215$ customers.

24. D
As the lawn is square , the length of one side will be the square root of the area. $\sqrt{62,500} = 250$ meters. So, the perimeter is found by 4 times the length of the side of the square:

$250•4 = 1000$ meters.

Since each meter costs $5.5, the total cost of the fence will be $1000•5.5 = \$5,500$.

25. B
$5n + (19 – 2) = 67$, $5n + 17 = 67$, $5n = 67 -17$, $5n = 50$, $n = 50/5 = 10$

26. B

Day	Absent	Present	%
Monday	5	40	88.88%
Tuesday	9	36	80.00%
Wednesday	4	41	91.11%
Thursday	10	35	77.77%
Friday	6	39	86.66%

Sum of the percent attendance is 424.42. Divide by 5 for the average, 424.42/5 = 84.884. Round up to 85%.

27. B
The distribution is done in three different rates and amounts:

$6.4 per 20 kilograms to 15 shops ... 20•15 = 300 kilograms distributed

$3.4 per 10 kilograms to 12 shops ... 10•12 = 120 kilograms distributed

550 - (300 + 120) = 550 - 420 = 130 kilograms left. This amount is distributed by 5 kilogram portions. So, this means that there are 130/5 = 26 shops.

$1.8 per 130 kilograms.

We need to find the amount he earned overall these distributions.

$6.4 per 20 kilograms : 6.4•15 = $96 for 300 kilograms

$3.4 per 10 kilograms : 3.4•12 = $40.8 for 120 kilograms

$1.8 per 5 kilograms : 1.8•26 = $46.8 for 130 kilograms

So, he earned 96 + 40.8 + 46.8 = $ 183.6

The total distribution cost is given as $10

The profit is found by: Money earned - money spent ... It is important to remember that he bought 550 kilograms of potatoes for $165 at the beginning:

Profit = 183.6 - 10 - 165 = $8.6

28. B
We check the fractions taking place in the question. We see that there is a "half" (that is 1/2) and 3/7. So, we multiply the denominators of these fractions to decide how to name the total money. We say that Mr. Johnson has 14x at the beginning; he gives half of this, meaning 7x, to his family. $250 to his landlord. He has 3/7 of his money left. 3/7 of 14x is equal to:

$14x \cdot (3/7) = 6x$

So,

Spent money is: 7x + 250

Unspent money is: 6x

Total money is: 14x

We write an equation: total money = spent money + unspent money

$14x = 7x + 250 + 6x$

$14x - 7x - 6x = 250$

$x = 250$

We are asked to find the total money that is 14x:

$14x = 14 \cdot 250 = \$3500$

29. A
The probability that the 1st ball drawn is red = 4/11
The probability that the 2nd ball drawn is green = 5/10
The combined probability will then be 4/11 X 5/10 = 20/110 = 2/11

30. D
First calculate total square feet, which is $15 \cdot 24 = 360$ ft^2. Next, convert this value to square yards, (1 yards^2 = 9 ft^2) which is 360/9 = 40 yards^2. At $0.50 per square yard, the total cost is $40 \cdot 0.50 = \$20$.

Section III English

1. A
The third conditional is used for talking about an unreal situation (a situation that did not happen) in the past. For example, "If I had studied harder, [if clause] I would have passed the exam" [main clause]. This has the same meaning as, "I failed the exam, because I didn't study hard enough."

2. A
Use a plural verb form for two subjects linked by "and."

3. B
In double negative sentences, one negative is replaced with "any."

4. C
"It's" is a contraction for it is or it has. "Its" is a possessive pronoun.

5. A
When two subjects are linked by "with" or "as well," use the verb form that matches the first subject.

6. A
The sentence requires the past perfect "has always been known." This is the only grammatically correct choice.

7. C
The superlative, "hottest," is used when expressing a temperature greater than that of anything to which it is being compared.

8. D
When comparing two items, use "the taller." When comparing more than two items, use "the tallest."

9. B
The past perfect form is used to describe an event that occurred in the past and prior to another event. Here there are two things that happened, both of them in the past, and something the person wanted to do.

Event 1: Kiss came to town
Event 2: All the tickets sold out
What I wanted to do: Buy a ticket

The events are arranged:
When KISS came to town, all the tickets **had been sold out** before I could buy one.

10. A
The subject is "rules" so the present tense plural form, "are," is used to agree with "realize."

11. A
"Who" is correct because the question uses an active construction. "To whom was first place given?" is a passive construction.

12. D
"Which" is correct, because the files are objects and not people.

13. B
Use a singular verb with either, each, neither, everyone and many.

14. D
Maintenance is the correct spelling.

15. C
Humorous is the correct spelling.

16. A
Mathematics is the correct spelling.

17. A
Use a comma to separate phrases.

18. A
The Sahara Desert is a proper name so capitalized. The names of countries, ie Africa are capitalized.

19. A
'She' is the simple subject of this sentence.

20. A
The simple predicate is 'studied long and hard.' The predicate of a sentence is the action performed by the subject.

21. B
This is an interrogative sentence.

22. C
It is not necessary to say the fish came from the topics, since we already know they are tropical.

23. B
The correct sentence is
Historians have been guessing for more than 100 years the doctor was a woman.

Here the phrase 'for more than 100 years' refers to how long historians have been guessing, and not to how long the doctor has been a woman.

24. B
Use a comma separates independent clauses. None of us wants to go to the party, not even if there will be live music.

25. A
This is an example where a comma appears before 'and,' but is disambiguating. Without the comma, the sentence would be "I own two dogs, a cat named Jeffrey and Henry, the goldfish." This means there is a cat named Jeffrey and Henry, and a goldfish with no name mentioned. The comma appears to show the distinction.

I own two dogs, a cat named Jeffrey, and Henry, the goldfish.

26. B
President is not capitalized unless used with a name as in, President Obama.

27. B
'Jumped' is a verb. Verbs describe an action, state, or occurrence.

28. B
A confrontation is a head-on conflict, so a direct confrontation is redundant.

29. D
Pesticide: NOUN a substance, usually synthetic although sometimes biological, used to kill or contain the activities of pests.

30. B
Hormones: NOUN any substance produced by one tissue and conveyed by the bloodstream to another to effect physiological activity.

Section IV – Science

1. A
Phenotype refers to observed properties of an organism and genotype refers to the genes of an organism.

2. A
A solution with a pH value of greater than 7 is base.

3. A
Eukaryotic and prokaryotic cells are both organelles.

4. C
Homologous is being inherited by the organisms' common ancestors. An example would be feathers and hair—both of which were structures that shared a common ancestral trait.

5. C
The manner in which instructions for building proteins, the basic structural molecules of living material are written in the DNA is a **genetic code**.

6. C
A gene is a unit of inherited material, encoded by a strand of DNA and transcribed by RNA.

7. D
All these statements are correct.

    a. During meiosis, the number of chromosomes in the cell are halved.

    b. Meiosis only occurs in eukaryotic cells.

    c. Meiosis is the part of the life cycle that involves sexual reproduction.

8. A Carrying capacity
An area's carrying capacity is the maximum number of animals of a given species that area can support during the harshest part of the year.

9. B
Diverticulitis is a pouch in the large intestine becomes inflamed.

10. A
Detection of pathogens can be complicated because they evolve so quickly.

11. A
Photosynthesis is the process by which plants and other photoautotrophs generate carbohydrates and oxygen from carbon dioxide, water, and light energy in chloroplasts.

12. C
Mutations in DNA sequences usually occur spontaneously is false.

Note: Mutations result when the DNA polymerase makes a mistake, which happens about once every 100,000,000 bases. Actually, the number of mistakes that remain incorporated into the DNA is even lower than this because cells contain special DNA repair proteins that fix many of the mistakes in the DNA that are caused by mutagens. The repair proteins see which nucleotides are paired incorrectly, and then change the wrong base to the right one. [14]

13. A

Starting with the weakest, the fundamental forces of nature in order of strength are, Gravity, Weak nuclear force, Electromagnetic force, Strong nuclear force.

Note: Although gravitational force is the weakest of the four, it acts over great distances. Electromagnetic force is of order 10^{39} times stronger than gravity. [15]

14. A

Precision, which refers to the repeatability of measurement, does not require knowledge of the correct or true value.

15. A

Artificial selection is a process where desirable traits are systematically bred.

16. C

Condensation is not an example of vaporization. Boiling and evaporation are both examples of vaporization. Condensation is the process by which matter transitions from a gas into a liquid.

17. B

The periodic table is a tabular display of the chemical elements, organized by their atomic numbers, electron configurations, and recurring chemical properties.

18. A

In terms of the scientific method, the term observation refers to the act of noticing or perceiving something and/or recording a fact or occurrence.

19. B

Kinetic energy is the energy of a body that results from motion while potential energy is the energy possessed by an object by virtue of its position or state, e.g., as in a compressed spring.

20. A

A life cycle is the sequence of developmental stages through which members of a given species must pass.

21. A
The cell membrane is a biological membrane that separates the interior of all cells from the outside environment. The cell membrane is selectively permeable to ions and organic molecules and controls the movement of substances in and out of cells. [16]

22. D
Relative position. Ranks include Domain, Kingdom, Phylum, Class, Order, Family, Genus, and Species.

23. D
A Standard deviation is a statistic used as a measure of the dispersion or variation in a distribution.

24. B
Substances that deactivate catalysts are called catalytic poisons.

25. B
Kinetic energy is the energy an object possesses due to its motion.

26. C
The interval of confidence around the measured value, such that the measured value is certain not to lie outside the stated interval refers to the **uncertainty** of that value.

27. D
Arteries carry oxygenated blood away from the heart, veins return oxygen-depleted blood to the heart, and capillaries are thin-walled blood vessels in which gas/ nutrient/ waste exchange occurs.

Note: An easy way to remember the difference between an artery and a vein is that Arteries carry Away from the heart.

28. B
The thoracic diaphragm, or simply the diaphragm, is a sheet of internal skeletal muscle that extends across the bottom of the rib cage. The diaphragm separates the thoracic cavity

(heart, lungs & ribs) from the abdominal cavity and performs an important function in respiration. [17]

29. D
Scientific classification. The two phrases are interchange-able, although the former seems to more accurately reflect the purpose of classification: to categorize biological units.

30. C
A recessive gene is not expressed as a trait unless inherited by both parents.

31. D
A scientific model is an approximation or simulation of a real system that omits all but the most essential variables of the system.

32. A
Neutrons are necessary within an atomic nucleus as they bind with protons via the nuclear force.

33. C
The following statement is false - Most enzymes are inor-ganic.

34. C
Acids are compounds that contain hydrogen and can dis-solve in water to release hydrogen ions into solution.

35. A
Genes determine individual hereditary characteristics.

36. A
The groups into which organisms are classified are called taxa and include, in order of size, Genus, Kingdom, Phylum/ division, Class, Order, and Family Species.

37. D
Digestion begins in the mouth.

38. A
The main components of the circulatory system are the

heart, veins and blood vessels.

39. D
An example of a pathogen that the immune system detects is a virus.

40. A
Chemical bonds are attractions between atoms that form chemical substances containing two or more atoms.

41. B
Cleansing food of impurities is not an example of a function of the stomach in digestion.

42. D
The exchange of oxygen for carbon dioxide takes place in the alveolar area of the lungs.

43. C
In chemistry, the number of protons in the nucleus of an atom is known as the atomic number, which determines the chemical element to which the atom belongs.

44. C
Natural selection is a process where biological traits become more or less common in a population.

45. A
Females have two X chromosomes and males have one X chromosome and one Y chromosome.

46. A
The immune system fight off disease by identifying and killing tumor cells and pathogens.

47. A
Water has two hydrogen atoms covalently bonded to one oxygen atom.

48. C
Choice C (Atomic theory explains temperature as the mo-

mentum of atoms.) is incorrect because atomic theory explains temperature as the motion of atoms (faster = hotter), not the momentum. The momentum of atoms explains the outward pressure that they exert.

Practice Test Questions Set 2

Section I – Reading

Questions: 42
Time: 45 Minutes

Section II – Math

Questions: 30
Time: 30 Minutes

Section III – English and Language Usage

Questions: 30
Time: 30 Minutes

Section IV – Science

Questions: 48
Time: 40 Minutes

The questions below are not the same as you will find on the HOBET® - that would be too easy! And nobody knows what the questions will be and they change all the time. Below are general questions that cover the same subject areas as the HOBET®. So, while the format and exact wording of the questions may differ slightly, and change from year to year, if you can answer the questions below, you will have no problem with the HOBET®.

For the best results, take these practice test questions as if it were the real exam. Set aside time when you will not be disturbed, and a location that is quiet and free of distractions. Read the instructions carefully, read each question carefully, and answer to the best of your ability.

You are given 209 minutes to complete the full HOBET® exam.

Use the bubble answer sheets provided. When you have completed the practice test questions, check your answer against the Answer Key and read the explanation provided.

Do not attempt more than one set of practice test questions in one day. After completing the first practice test, wait two or three days before attempting the second set of questions.

Section I – Reading Answer Sheet

1. (A) (B) (C) (D)
2. (A) (B) (C) (D)
3. (A) (B) (C) (D)
4. (A) (B) (C) (D)
5. (A) (B) (C) (D)
6. (A) (B) (C) (D)
7. (A) (B) (C) (D)
8. (A) (B) (C) (D)
9. (A) (B) (C) (D)
10. (A) (B) (C) (D)
11. (A) (B) (C) (D)
12. (A) (B) (C) (D)
13. (A) (B) (C) (D)
14. (A) (B) (C) (D)
15. (A) (B) (C) (D)
16. (A) (B) (C) (D)
17. (A) (B) (C) (D)

18. (A) (B) (C) (D)
19. (A) (B) (C) (D)
20. (A) (B) (C) (D)
21. (A) (B) (C) (D)
22. (A) (B) (C) (D)
23. (A) (B) (C) (D)
24. (A) (B) (C) (D)
25. (A) (B) (C) (D)
26. (A) (B) (C) (D)
27. (A) (B) (C) (D)
28. (A) (B) (C) (D)
29. (A) (B) (C) (D)
30. (A) (B) (C) (D)
31. (A) (B) (C) (D)
32. (A) (B) (C) (D)
33. (A) (B) (C) (D)
34. (A) (B) (C) (D)

35. (A) (B) (C) (D)
36. (A) (B) (C) (D)
37. (A) (B) (C) (D)
38. (A) (B) (C) (D)
39. (A) (B) (C) (D)
40. (A) (B) (C) (D)
41. (A) (B) (C) (D)
42. (A) (B) (C) (D)

Section II – Math – Answer Sheet

1. Ⓐ Ⓑ Ⓒ Ⓓ 11. Ⓐ Ⓑ Ⓒ Ⓓ 21. Ⓐ Ⓑ Ⓒ Ⓓ

2. Ⓐ Ⓑ Ⓒ Ⓓ 12. Ⓐ Ⓑ Ⓒ Ⓓ 22. Ⓐ Ⓑ Ⓒ Ⓓ

3. Ⓐ Ⓑ Ⓒ Ⓓ 13. Ⓐ Ⓑ Ⓒ Ⓓ 23. Ⓐ Ⓑ Ⓒ Ⓓ

4. Ⓐ Ⓑ Ⓒ Ⓓ 14. Ⓐ Ⓑ Ⓒ Ⓓ 24. Ⓐ Ⓑ Ⓒ Ⓓ

5. Ⓐ Ⓑ Ⓒ Ⓓ 15. Ⓐ Ⓑ Ⓒ Ⓓ 25. Ⓐ Ⓑ Ⓒ Ⓓ

6. Ⓐ Ⓑ Ⓒ Ⓓ 16. Ⓐ Ⓑ Ⓒ Ⓓ 26. Ⓐ Ⓑ Ⓒ Ⓓ

7. Ⓐ Ⓑ Ⓒ Ⓓ 17. Ⓐ Ⓑ Ⓒ Ⓓ 27. Ⓐ Ⓑ Ⓒ Ⓓ

8. Ⓐ Ⓑ Ⓒ Ⓓ 18. Ⓐ Ⓑ Ⓒ Ⓓ 28. Ⓐ Ⓑ Ⓒ Ⓓ

9. Ⓐ Ⓑ Ⓒ Ⓓ 19. Ⓐ Ⓑ Ⓒ Ⓓ 29. Ⓐ Ⓑ Ⓒ Ⓓ

10. Ⓐ Ⓑ Ⓒ Ⓓ 20. Ⓐ Ⓑ Ⓒ Ⓓ 30. Ⓐ Ⓑ Ⓒ Ⓓ

Section III – English and Language Usage Answer Sheet

1. (A) (B) (C) (D)   11. (A) (B) (C) (D)   21. (A) (B) (C) (D)

2. (A) (B) (C) (D)   12. (A) (B) (C) (D)   22. (A) (B) (C) (D)

3. (A) (B) (C) (D)   13. (A) (B) (C) (D)   23. (A) (B) (C) (D)

4. (A) (B) (C) (D)   14. (A) (B) (C) (D)   24. (A) (B) (C) (D)

5. (A) (B) (C) (D)   15. (A) (B) (C) (D)   25. (A) (B) (C) (D)

6. (A) (B) (C) (D)   16. (A) (B) (C) (D)   26. (A) (B) (C) (D)

7. (A) (B) (C) (D)   17. (A) (B) (C) (D)   27. (A) (B) (C) (D)

8. (A) (B) (C) (D)   18. (A) (B) (C) (D)   28. (A) (B) (C) (D)

9. (A) (B) (C) (D)   19. (A) (B) (C) (D)   29. (A) (B) (C) (D)

10. (A) (B) (C) (D)   20. (A) (B) (C) (D)   30. (A) (B) (C) (D)

Practice the HOBET®

Section IV – Science Answer Sheet

1. (A) (B) (C) (D)
2. (A) (B) (C) (D)
3. (A) (B) (C) (D)
4. (A) (B) (C) (D)
5. (A) (B) (C) (D)
6. (A) (B) (C) (D)
7. (A) (B) (C) (D)
8. (A) (B) (C) (D)
9. (A) (B) (C) (D)
10. (A) (B) (C) (D)
11. (A) (B) (C) (D)
12. (A) (B) (C) (D)
13. (A) (B) (C) (D)
14. (A) (B) (C) (D)
15. (A) (B) (C) (D)
16. (A) (B) (C) (D)
17. (A) (B) (C) (D)

18. (A) (B) (C) (D)
19. (A) (B) (C) (D)
20. (A) (B) (C) (D)
21. (A) (B) (C) (D)
22. (A) (B) (C) (D)
23. (A) (B) (C) (D)
24. (A) (B) (C) (D)
25. (A) (B) (C) (D)
26. (A) (B) (C) (D)
27. (A) (B) (C) (D)
28. (A) (B) (C) (D)
29. (A) (B) (C) (D)
30. (A) (B) (C) (D)
31. (A) (B) (C) (D)
32. (A) (B) (C) (D)
33. (A) (B) (C) (D)
34. (A) (B) (C) (D)

35. (A) (B) (C) (D)
36. (A) (B) (C) (D)
37. (A) (B) (C) (D)
38. (A) (B) (C) (D)
39. (A) (B) (C) (D)
40. (A) (B) (C) (D)
41. (A) (B) (C) (D)
42. (A) (B) (C) (D)
43. (A) (B) (C) (D)
44. (A) (B) (C) (D)
45. (A) (B) (C) (D)
46. (A) (B) (C) (D)
47. (A) (B) (C) (D)
48. (A) (B) (C) (D)
49. (A) (B) (C) (D)
50. (A) (B) (C) (D)

Section I - Reading

Questions 1-4 refer to the following passage.

Passage 1 - The Respiratory System

The respiratory system's function is to allow oxygen exchange through all parts of the body. The anatomy or structure of the exchange system, and the uses of the exchanged gases, varies depending on the organism. In humans and other mammals, for example, the anatomical features of the respiratory system include airways, lungs, and the respiratory muscles. Molecules of oxygen and carbon dioxide are passively exchanged, by diffusion, between the gaseous external environment and the blood. This exchange process occurs in the alveolar region of the lungs.

Other animals, such as insects, have respiratory systems with very simple anatomical features, and in amphibians even the skin plays a vital role in gas exchange. Plants also have respiratory systems but the direction of gas exchange can be opposite to that of animals.

The respiratory system can also be divided into physiological, or functional, zones. These include the conducting zone (the region for gas transport from the outside atmosphere to just above the alveoli), the transitional zone, and the respiratory zone (the alveolar region where gas exchange occurs). [18]

1. What can we infer from the first paragraph in this passage?

    a. Human and mammal respiratory systems are the same.

    b. The lungs are an important part of the respiratory system.

    c. The respiratory system varies in different mammals.

    d. Oxygen and carbon dioxide are passive exchanged by the respiratory system.

2. What is the process by which molecules of oxygen and carbon dioxide are passively exchanged?

    a. Transfusion

    b. Affusion

    c. Diffusion

    d. Respiratory confusion

3. What organ plays an important role in gas exchange in amphibians?

    a. The skin

    b. The lungs

    c. The gills

    d. The mouth

4. What are the three physiological zones of the respiratory system?

    a. Conducting, transitional, respiratory zones

    b. Redacting, transitional, circulatory zones

    c. Conducting, circulatory, inhibiting zones

    d. Transitional, inhibiting, conducting zones

Questions 5 - 8 refer to the following passage.

The Civil War

The Civil War began on April 12, 1861. The first shots of the Civil War were fired in Fort Sumter, South Carolina. Note that even though more American lives were lost in the Civil War than in any other war, not one person died on that first day. The war began because eleven Southern states seceded from the Union and tried to start their own government, The Confederate States of America.

Why did the states secede? The issue of slavery was a primary cause of the Civil War. The eleven southern states relied heavily on their slaves to foster their farming and plantation lifestyles. The northern states, many of whom had already abolished slavery, did not think that the southern states should have slaves. The north wanted to free all the slaves and President Lincoln's goal was to both end slavery and preserve the Union. He had Congress declared war on the Confederacy on April 14, 1862. For four long, blood soaked years, the North and South fought.

From 1861 to mid 1863, it seemed as if the South would win this war. However, on July 1, 1863, an epic three day battle was waged on a field in Gettysburg, Pennsylvania. Gettysburg is remembered for being the bloodiest battle in American history. At the end of the three days, the North turned the tide of the war in their favor. The North then went onto dominate the South for the remainder of the war. Most well remembered might be General Sherman's "March to The Sea," where he famously led the Union Army through Georgia and the Carolinas, burning and destroying everything in their path.

In 1865, the Union army invaded and captured the Confederate capital of Richmond Virginia. Robert E. Lee, leader of the Confederacy surrendered to General Ulysses S. Grant, leader of the Union forces, on April 9, 1865. The Civil War was over, and the Union was preserved.

5. What does the word secede most nearly mean?

    a. To break away from

    b. To accomplish

    c. To join

    d. To lose

6. Which of the following statements summarizes a FACT from the passage?

a. Congress declared war and then the Battle of Fort Sumter began.

b. Congress declared war after shots were fired at Fort Sumter.

c. President Lincoln was pro slavery

d. President Lincoln was at Fort Sumter with Congress

7. Which event finally led the Confederacy to surrender?

a. The battle of Gettysburg

b. The battle of Bull Run

c. The invasion of the confederate capital of Richmond

d. Sherman's March to the Sea

8. The word abolish as used in this passage most nearly means?

a. To ban

b. To polish

c. To support

d. To destroy

Questions 9 – 11 refer to the following passage.

Passage 2 – Mythology

The main characters in myths are usually gods or super-natural heroes. As sacred stories, rulers and priests have traditionally endorsed their myths and as a result, myths have a close link with religion and politics. In the society where a myth originates, the natives believe the myth is a true account of the remote past. In fact, many societies have two categories of traditional narrative—(1) "true stories," or myths, and (2) "false stories," or fables.

Myths generally take place during a primordial age, when the world was still young, before achieving its current form. These stories explain how the world gained its current form and why the culture developed its customs, institutions, and taboos. Closely related to myth are legend and folktale. Myths, legends, and folktales are different types of traditional stories. Unlike myths, folktales can take place at any time and any place, and the natives do not usually consider them true or sacred. Legends, on the other hand, are similar to myths in that many people have traditionally considered them true. Legends take place in a more recent time, when the world was much as it is today. In addition, legends generally feature humans as their main characters, whereas myths have superhuman characters. [19]

9. We can infer from this passage that

a. Folktales took place in a time far past, before civilization covered the earth.

b. Humankind uses myth to explain how the world was created.

c. Myths revolve around gods or supernatural beings; the local community usually accepts these stories as not true.

d. The only difference between a myth and a legend is the time setting of the story.

10. The main purpose of this passage is

a. To distinguish between many types of traditional stories, and explain the background of some traditional story categories.

b. To determine whether myths and legends might be true accounts of history.

c. To show the importance of folktales how these traditional stories made life more bearable in harder times.

d. None of the Above.

11. How are folktales different from myths?

a. Folktales and myth are the same.

b. Folktales are not true and generally not sacred and take place anytime.

c. Myths are not true and generally not sacred and take place anytime.

d. Folktales explained the formation of the world and myths do not.

Questions 12 refers to the following table of contents.

Getting Started

12. Based on the partial table of contents above, what is this book about?

a. How to answer multiple choice questions

b. Different types of multiple choice questions

c. How to write a test

d. None of the above

Questions 13 - 16 refer to the following passage.

Passage 3 – Myths, Legend and Folklore

Cultural historians draw a distinction between myth, legend and folktale simply as a way to group traditional stories. However, in many cultures, drawing a sharp line between myths and legends is not that simple. Instead of dividing their traditional stories into myths, legends, and folktales, some cultures divide them into two categories. The first category roughly corresponds with folktales, and the second is one that combines myths and legends. Similarly, we cannot always separate myths from folktales. One society might consider a story true, making it a myth. Another society may believe the story is fiction, which makes it a folktale. In fact, when a myth loses its status as part of a religious system, it often takes on traits more typical of folktales, with its formerly divine characters now appearing as human heroes, giants, or fairies. Myth, legend, and folktale are only a few of the categories of traditional stories. Other categories include anecdotes and some kinds of jokes. Traditional stories, in turn, are only one category within the larger category of folklore, which also includes items such as gestures, costumes, and music. [19]

13. The main idea of this passage is that

a. Myths, fables, and folktales are not the same thing, and each describes a specific type of story.

b. Traditional stories can be categorized in different ways by different people.

c. Cultures use myths for religious purposes, and when this is no longer true, the people forget and discard these myths.

d. Myths can never become folk tales, because one is true, and the other is false.

14. The terms myth and legend are

a. Categories that are synonymous with true and false.

b. Categories that group traditional stories according to certain characteristics.

c. Interchangeable, because both terms mean a story that is passed down from generation to generation.

d. Meant to distinguish between a story that involves a hero and a cultural message and a story meant only to entertain.

15. Traditional story categories not only include myths and legends, but

> a. Can also include gestures, since some cultures passed these down before the written and spoken word.
>
> b. In addition, folklore refers to stories involving fables and fairy tales.
>
> c. These story categories can also include folk music and traditional dress.
>
> d. Traditional stories themselves are a part of the larger category of folklore, which may also include costumes, gestures, and music.

16. This passage shows that

> a. There is a distinct difference between a myth and a legend, both are folktales.
>
> b. Myths are folktales, but folktales are not myths.
>
> c. Myths, legends, and folktales play an important part in tradition and the past, and are a rich and colorful part of history.

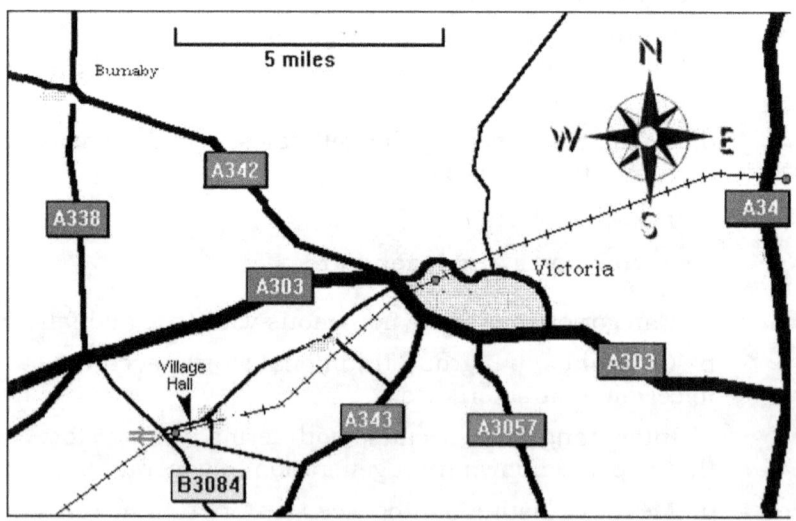

17. Approximately how far is Victoria to Burnaby?

a. About 10 miles

b. About 5 miles

c. About 15 miles

d. About 20 miles

18. How is the Village Hall from Victoria?

a. About 10 miles

b. About 5 miles

c. About 15 miles

d. About 20 miles

Questions 19 - 23 refer to the following passage.

A Day That Will Live in Infamy! Attack on Pearl Harbor

In 1941, the world was at war. The United States was trying very hard to keep itself out of the conflict. In Europe, the countries of Germany and Italy had formed an alliance to expand their land and territory. Germany had already taken over Poland, Denmark, and parts of France. They were heading next toward England and due to all the fighting in Europe, there were battles taking place as far south as North Africa, where the German and Italian armies were fighting the British.

This got even worse when the Asian nation of Japan formed an alliance with Germany and Italy. Together, the three countries called themselves, the AXIS. Now, the war was in the Pacific as well as in Europe and Northern Africa. Many Americans thought that perhaps now was the time for the United States to join with its ally, Great Britain and stop the Axis from taking over more regions of the world.

In 1941, Franklin Roosevelt was President of the United States. His fear at the time was that Japan would try to take over many countries in Asia. He did not want to see that happen, so he moved some of the United States warships that had been stationed in San Diego, to the military base at Pearl Harbor, in Honolulu, Hawaii.

Japan quietly plotted their attack. They waited until the early hours of the morning on Sunday, December 7, 1941. Then, 350 Japanese war plans began to drop bombs on the U.S. ships at Pearl Harbor.

The first bombs fell at 7:48 am and a mere 90 minutes later, the attack was over. Pearl Harbor was decimated. 8 battleships were damaged. Eleven ships were sunk and 300 U.S. planes were destroyed. Most devastating was the loss of life 2,400 U.S. military members was killed in the attack and 1, 282 were injured.

President Roosevelt addressed the country via the radio and said "Today is a day that will live in infamy." He asked Congress to declare war on Japan. War was declared on Japan on December 8th and on Germany and Italy on December 11th. The United States had entered World War Two.

19. After reading the passage, what can we infer the word infamy means?

    a. Famous

    b. Remembered in a good way

    c. Remembered in a bad way

    d. Easily forgotten

20. What three countries formed the Axis?

    a. Italy, England, Germany

    b. United States, England, Italy

    c. Germany, Japan, Italy

    d. Germany, Japan, United States

21. What do you think was President Roosevelt's reason for moving warships to Pearl Harbor?

a. He feared Japan would bomb San Diego

b. He knew Japan was going to attack Pearl Harbor

c. He was planning to attack Japan

d. He wanted to try to protect Asian countries from Japanese takeover

22. Why do you think Japan chose a Sunday morning at 7:48 am for their attack?

a. They knew the military slept late

b. There is a law against bombing countries on a Sunday

c. They wanted the attack to catch people by surprise

d. That was the only free time they had to attack.

Questions 23 - 26 refer to the following passage.

The Winged Victory of Samothrace: the Statue of the Gods

Students who read about the "Winged Victory of Samothrace" probably won't be able to picture what the statue looks like. However, almost anyone who knows little about statues will recognize it when they see it: it is the statue of a winged woman who does not have arms or a head. Even the most famous pieces of art may be recognized by sight but not by name.

This iconic statue is of the Greek goddess Nike, who represented victory and was called Victoria by the Romans. The statue is sometimes called the "Nike of Samothrace." She was often displayed in Greek art as driving a chariot, and her speed or efficiency with the chariot may be what her wings symbolize. It is said that the statue was created around 200 BCE to celebrate a battle that was won at sea. Archaeologists and art historians believe the statue may have originally been part of a temple or other building, even one of the most important temples, Megaloi Theoi, just as many statues were used during that time.

"Winged Victory" does indeed appear to have had arms and a head when it was originally created, and it is unclear why they were removed or lost. Indeed, they have never been discovered, even with all the excavation that has taken place. Many speculate that one of her arms was raised and put to her mouth, as though she was shouting or calling out, which is consistent with the idea of her as a war figure. If the missing pieces were ever to be found, they might give Greek and art historians more of an idea of what Nike represented or how the statue was used.

Learning about pieces of art through details like these can help students remember time frames or locations, as well as learn about the people who occupied them.

23. The author's title says the statue is "of the Gods" because

> a. the statue is very beautiful and even a god would find it beautiful
>
> b. the statue is of a Greek goddess, and gods were of primary importance to the Greek
>
> c. Nike lead the gods into war
>
> d. the statues were used at the temple of the gods and so it belonged to them

24. The third paragraph states that

> a. the statue is related to war and was probably broken apart by foreign soldiers
>
> b. the arms and head of the statue cannot be found because all the excavation has taken place
>
> c. speculations have been made about what the entire statue looked like and what it symbolized
>
> d. the statue has no arms or head because the sculptor lost them

25. The author's main purpose in writing this passage is to

   a. demonstrate that art and culture are related and one can teach us about the other

   b. persuade readers to become archeologists and find the missing pieces of the statue

   c. teach readers about the Greek goddess Nike

   d. to teach readers the name of a statue they probably recognize

26. The author specifies the indirect audience as "students" because

   a. it is probably a student who is taking this test

   b. most young people don't know much about art yet, and most young people are students

   c. students read more than people who are not students

   d. the passage is based on a discussion of what we can learn about culture from art

Questions 27 - 29 refer to the following passage.

Lowest Price Guarantee

Get it for less. Guaranteed!

ABC Electric will beat any advertised price by 10% of the difference.

   1) If you find a lower advertised price, we will beat it by 10% of the difference.

   2) If you find a lower advertised price within 30 days* of your purchase we will beat it by 10% of the difference.

   3) If our own price is reduced within 30 days* of your purchase, bring in your receipt and we will refund the difference.

*14 days for computers, monitors, printers, laptops, tablets, cellular & wireless devices, home security products, projectors, camcorders, digital cameras, radar detectors, portable DVD players, DJ and pro-audio equipment, and air conditioners.

27. I bought a radar detector 15 days ago and saw an ad for the same model only cheaper. Can I get 10% of the difference refunded?

a. Yes. Since it is less than 30 days, you can get 10% of the difference refunded.

b. No. Since it is more than 14 days, you cannot get 10% of the difference re-funded.

c. It depends on the cashier.

d. Yes. You can get the difference refunded.

28. I bought a flat-screen TV for $500 10 days ago and found an advertisement for the same TV, at another store, on sale for $400. How much will ABC refund under this guarantee?

a. $100

b. $110

c. $10

d. $400

29. What is the purpose of this passage?

a. To inform

b. To educate

c. To persuade

d. To entertain

Questions 30 - 33 refer to the following passage.

Ways Characters Communicate in Theater

Playwrights give their characters voices in a way that gives depth and added meaning to what happens on stage during their play. There are different types of speech in scripts that allow characters to talk with themselves, with other characters, and even with the audience.

It is very unique to theater that characters may talk "to themselves." When characters do this, the speech they give is called a soliloquy. Soliloquies are usually poetic, introspective, moving, and can tell audience members about the feelings, motivations, or suspicions of an individual character without that character having to reveal them to other characters on stage. "To be or not to be" is a famous soliloquy given by Hamlet as he considers difficult but important themes, such as life and death.

The most common type of communication in plays is when one character is speaking to another or a group of other characters. This is generally called dialogue, but can also be called monologue if one character speaks without being interrupted for a long time. It is not necessarily the most important type of communication, but it is the most common because the plot of the play cannot really progress without it.

Lastly, and most unique to theater (although it has been used somewhat in film) is when a character speaks directly to the audience. This is called an aside, and scripts usually specifically direct actors to do this. Asides are usually comical, an inside joke between the character and the audience, and very short. The actor will usually face the audience when delivering them, even if it's for a moment, so the audience can recognize this move as an aside.

All three of these types of communication are important to the art of theater, and have been perfected by famous playwrights like Shakespeare. Understanding these types of communication can help an audience member grasp what is artful about the script and action of a play.

30. According to the passage, characters in plays communicate to

    a. move the plot forward

    b. show the private thoughts and feelings of one character

    c. make the audience laugh

    d. add beauty and artistry to the play

31. When Hamlet delivers "To be or not to be," he can most likely be described as

    a. solitary

    b. thoughtful

    c. dramatic

    d. hopeless

32. The author uses parentheses to punctuate "although it has been used somewhat in film"

    a. to show that films are less important

    b. instead of using commas so that the sentence is not interrupted

    c. because parenthesis help separate details that are not as important

    d. to show that films are not as artistic

33. It can be understood that by the phrase "give their characters voices," the author means that

    a. playwrights are generous

    b. playwrights are changing the sound or meaning of characters' voices to fit what they had in mind

    c. dialogue is important in creating characters

    d. playwrights may be the parent of one of their actors and give them their voice

Questions 34 - 37 refer to the following passage.

Passage 7 - The Circulatory System

The circulatory system is an organ system that passes nutrients (such as amino acids and electrolytes), gases, hormones, and blood cells to and from cells in the body to help fight diseases and help stabilize body temperature and pH levels.

The circulatory system may be seen strictly as a blood distribution network, but some consider the circulatory system as composed of the cardiovascular system, which distributes blood, and the lymphatic system, which distributes lymph. While humans, as well as other vertebrates, have a closed cardiovascular system (meaning that the blood never leaves the network of arteries, veins and capillaries), some invertebrate groups have an open cardiovascular system. The most primitive animal phyla lack circulatory systems. The lymphatic system, on the other hand, is an open system.

Two types of fluids move through the circulatory system: blood and lymph. The blood, heart, and blood vessels form the cardiovascular system. The lymph, the lymph nodes, and lymph vessels form the lymphatic system. The cardiovascular system and the lymphatic system collectively make up the circulatory system.

The main components of the human cardiovascular system are the heart and the blood vessels. It includes: the pulmonary circulation, a "loop" through the lungs where blood is oxygenated; and the systemic circulation, a "loop" through the rest of the body to provide oxygenated blood. An average adult contains five to six quarts (roughly 4.7 to 5.7 liters) of blood, which consists of plasma, red blood cells, white blood cells, and platelets. Also, the digestive system works with the circulatory system to provide the nutrients the system needs to keep the heart pumping. [20]

34. What can we infer from the first paragraph?

a. An important purpose of the circulatory system is that of fighting diseases.

b. The most important function of the circulatory system is to give the person energy.

c. The least important function of the circulatory system is that of growing skin cells.

d. The entire purpose of the circulatory system is not known.

35. Do humans have an open or closed circulatory system?

a. Open

b. Closed

c. Usually open, though sometimes closed

d. Usually closed, though sometimes open

36. Besides blood, what two components form the cardiovascular system?

a. The heart and the lungs

b. The lungs and the veins

c. The heart and the blood vessels

d. The blood vessels and the nerves

37. Which system, along with the circulatory system, helps provide nutrients to keep the human heart pumping?

a. The skeletal system

b. The digestive system

c. The immune system

d. The nervous system

Questions 38 - 41 refer to the following passage.

Passage 8 - Blood

Blood is a specialized bodily fluid that delivers nutrients and oxygen to the body's cells and transports waste products away.

In vertebrates, blood consists of blood cells suspended in a liquid called blood plasma. Plasma, which comprises 55% of blood fluid, is mostly water (90% by volume), and contains dissolved proteins, glucose, mineral ions, hormones, carbon dioxide, platelets and the blood cells themselves.

Blood cells are mainly red blood cells (also called RBCs or erythrocytes) and white blood cells, including leukocytes and platelets. Red blood cells are the most abundant cells, and contain an iron-containing protein called hemoglobin that transports oxygen through the body.

The pumping action of the heart circulates blood around the body through blood vessels. In animals with lungs, arterial blood carries oxygen from inhaled air to the tissues of the body, and venous blood carries carbon dioxide, a waste product of metabolism produced by cells, from the tissues to the lungs to be exhaled. [21]

38. What can we infer from the first paragraph in this passage?

   a. Blood is responsible for transporting oxygen to the cells.

   b. Blood is only red when it reaches the outside the body.

   c. Each person has about six pints of blood.

   d. Blood's true function was only learned in the last century.

39. What liquid are blood cells suspended?

    a. Plasma

    b. Water

    c. Liquid nitrogen

    d. A mixture consisting largely of human milk

40. Which of these is not contained in blood plasma?

    a. Hormones

    b. Mineral ions

    c. Calcium

    d. Glucose

41. Which body part exhales carbon dioxide after venous blood has carried it from body tissues?

    a. The lungs

    b. The skin cells

    c. The bowels

    d. The sweat glands

Question 42 refers to the following passage.

Passage 9 - The Human Skeleton

The human skeleton consists of both fused and individual bones supported and supplemented by ligaments, tendons, muscles and cartilage. It serves as a scaffold which supports organs, anchors muscles, and protects organs such as the brain, lungs and heart. The biggest bone in the body is the femur in the upper leg, and the smallest is the stapes bone in the middle ear. In an adult, the skeleton comprises around 14% of the total body weight, and half is water.

Fused bones include the pelvis and the cranium. Not all bones are interconnected directly: There are three bones in each middle ear called the ossicles that articulate only with each other. The thyroid bone, which is located in the neck, and serves as the point of attachment for the tongue, does not articulate with any other bones in the body, being supported by muscles and ligaments.

There are 206 bones in the adult human skeleton, which varies between individuals and with age - newborn babies have over 270 bones, some of which fuse together. These bones are organized into a longitudinal axis, the axial skeleton, to which the appendicular skeleton is attached. [22]

42. What is the main idea of this passage?

a. The human skeleton is an important and complicated system of the body.

b. There are 206 bones in the typical human body.

c. In a child, the skeleton represents 14% of the body weight.

d. Bones become more fragile as we age.

Section II – Math

1. Richard gives 's' amount of salary to each of his 'n' employees weekly. If he has 'x' amount of money, how many days he can employ these 'n' employees.

a. sx/7n

b. 7x/nx

c. nx/7s

d. 7x/ns

2. Translate the following into an equation: Five greater than 3 times a number.

    a. 3X + 5

    b. 5X + 3

    c. (5 + 3)X

    d. 5(3 + X)

3. What number is MMXIII?

    a. 2010

    b. 1990

    c. 2013

    d. 2012

4. Solve for x, when 5x + 21 = 66.

    a. 19

    b. 9

    c. 15

    d. 5

5. Write 765.3682 to the nearest 1000th.

    a. 765.368

    b. 765.36

    c. 765.3682

    d. 765.3

6. If Lynn can type a page in p minutes, what portion of the page can she do in 5 minutes?

    a. p/5

    b. p - 5

    c. p + 5

    d. 5/p

7. If Sally can paint a house in 4 hours, and John can paint the same house in 6 hours, how long will it take for both of to paint a house?

    a. 2 hours and 24 minutes

    b. 3 hours and 12 minutes

    c. 3 hours and 44 minutes

    d. 4 hours and 10 minutes

8. Employees of a discount appliance store receive an additional 20% off the lowest price on any item. If an employee purchases a dishwasher during a 15% off sale, how much will he pay if the dishwasher originally cost $450?

    a. $280.90

    b. $287.00

    c. $292.50

    d. $306.00

9. The sale price of a car is $12,590, which is 20% off the original price. What is the original price?

    a. $14,310.40

    b. $14,990.90

    c. $15,108.00

    d. $15,737.50

10. Express 25% as a fraction.

    a. 1/4

    b. 7/40

    c. 6/25

    d. 8/28

11. Express 125% as a decimal.

    a. .125

    b. 12.5

    c. 1.25

    d. 125

12. Express 24/56 as a reduced common fraction.

    a. 4/9

    b. 4/11

    c. 3/7

    d. 3/8

13. Express 71/1000 as a decimal.

    a. .71

    b. .0071

    c. .071

    d. 7.1

14. What number is in the ten thousandths place in 1.7389?

    a. 1

    b. 8

    c. 9

    d. 3

15. Simplify 6 3/5 – 4 4/5

    a. 1 4/5

    b. 2 3/5

    c. 2 9/5

    d. 1 1/5

16. The physician ordered 100 mg Ibuprofen/kg of body weight; on hand is 230 mg/tablet. The child weighs 50 lb. How many tablets will you give?

   a. 10 tablets

   b. 5 tablets

   c. 1 tablet

   d. 12 tablets

17. In a local election at polling station A, 945 voters cast their vote out of 1270 registered voters. At polling station B, 860 cast their vote out of 1050 registered voters and at station C, 1210 cast their vote out of 1440 registered voters. What is the total turnout from all three polling stations?

   a. 70%

   b. 74%

   c. 76%

   d. 80%

18. The physician ordered 600 mg ibuprofen; the pharmacy stocks 200 mg per tablet. How many tablets will you give?

   a. 3.5 tablets

   b. 2 tablets

   c. 5 tablets

   d. 3 tablets

19. The manager of a weaving factory estimates that if 10 machines run at 100% efficiency for 8 hours, they will produce 1450 meters of cloth. Due to some technical problems, 4 machines run of 95% efficiency and the remaining 6 at 90% efficiency. How many meters of cloth can these machines will produce in 8 hours?

    a. 1334 meters

    b. 1310 meters

    c. 1300 meters

    d. 1285 meters

20. Convert 60 feet to inches.

    a. 700 inches

    b. 600 inches

    c. 720 inches

    d. 1,800 inches

21. A box contains 7 black pencils and 28 blue ones. What is the ratio between the black and blue pens?

    a. 1:4

    b. 2:7

    c. 1:8

    d. 1:9

22. Convert 100 millimeters to centimeters.

    a. 10 centimeters

    b. 1,000 centimeters

    c. 1100 centimeters

    d. 50 centimeters

23. Convert 3 gallons to quarts.

    a. 15 quarts

    b. 6 quarts

    c. 12 quarts

    d. 32 quarts

24. A map uses a scale of 1:2,000 How much distance on the ground is 5.2 inches on the map if the scale is in inches?

    a. 100,400

    b. 10, 500

    c. 10,440

    d. 10,400

25. 0.05 ml. =

    a. 50 liters

    b. 0.00005 liters

    c. 5 liters

    d. 0.0005 liters

26. X% of 120 = 30. Solve for X.

    a. 15

    b. 12

    c. 4

    d. 25

27. Smith and Simon are playing a card game. Smith will win if a card drawn from a deck of 52 is either 7 or a diamond, and Simon will win if the drawn card is an even number. Which statement is more likely to be correct?

    a. Smith will win more games.

    b. Simon will win more games.

    c. They have same winning probability.

    d. A decision cannot be made from the provided data.

28. Convert .45 meters to centimeters

    a. 45

    b. 450

    c. 4.5

    d. .45

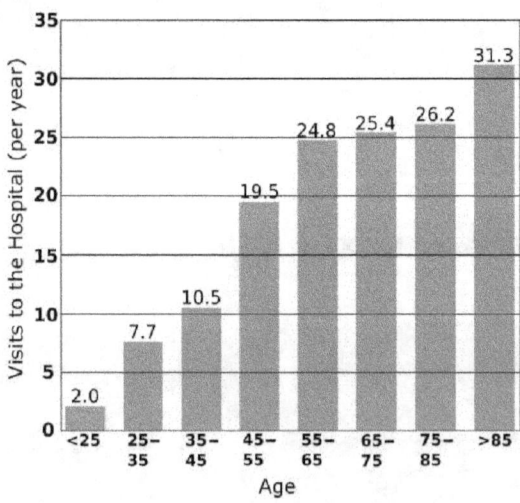

29. Consider the graph above.

How many hospital visits per year does a person aged 85 or more make?

  a. 26.2

  b. 31.3

  c. More than 31.3

  d. A decision cannot be made from this graph.

30. Based on this graph, how many visits per year do you expect a person that is 95 or older to make?

  a. 31.3 or more

  b. Less than 31.3

  c. 31.3

  d. A decision cannot be made from this graph.

Section III – English and Language Usage

1. Elaine promised to bring the camera _____ at the mall yesterday.

  a. by me

  b. with me

  c. at me

  d. to me

2. Last night, he _____ the sleeping bag down beside my mattress.

  a. lay

  b. laid

  c. lain

  d. has laid

3. I would have bought the shirt for you if

    a. I had known you liked it.

    b. I have known you liked it.

    c. I would know you liked it.

    d. I know you liked it.

4. Many believers still hope _____ proof of the existence of ghosts.

    a. two find

    b. to find

    c. to found

    d. to have been found

5. Choose the sentence with the correct grammar.

    a. The court summons was placed on his desk

    b. The court summons are placed on his desk

    c. The court summons were placed on his desk

    d. None of the above

6. To _____, Anne was on time for her math class.

    a. everybody's surprise

    b. every body's surprise

    c. everybodys surprise

    d. everybodys' surprise

7. As an added bonus, we got to see the orchestra warm up.

What part of this sentence is redundant?

    a. Added

    b. Bonus

    c. Warm up

    d. None of the above

8. If he _____ the textbook like he was supposed to, he would have known what was on the test.

   a. will have read

   b. shouldn't have read

   c. would have read

   d. had read

9. Following the tornado, telephone poles _____ all over the street.

   a. laid

   b. lied

   c. were lying

   d. were laying

10. In Edgar Allen Poe's _____ Edgar Allen Poe describes a man with a guilty conscience.

   a. short story, "The Tell-Tale Heart,"

   b. short story The Tell-Tale Heart,

   c. short story, The Tell-Tale Heart

   d. short story. "the Tell-Tale Heart,"

11. Billboards are considered an important part of advertising for big business, _____ by their critics.

   a. but, an eyesore;

   b. but, " an eyesore,"

   c. but an eyesore

   d. but-an eyesore-

12. I can never remember how to use those two common words, "sell," meaning to trade a product for money, or _____ meaning an event where products are traded for less money than usual.

    a. sale-

    b. "sale,"

    c. "sale

    d. "to sale,"

13. Choose the sentence with the correct grammar.

    a. Neither the teacher nor the students is left in class.

    b. Neither the teacher nor the students was left in class.

    c. Neither the teacher nor the students are left in class.

    d. None of the above.

14. The class just finished reading _____ a short story by Carl Stephenson about a plantation owner's battle with army ants.

    a. -"Leinengen versus the Ants,"

    b. Leinengen versus the Ants,

    c. "Leinengen versus the Ants,"

    d. Leinengen versus the Ants

15. After the car was fixed, it _____ again.

    a. ran good

    b. ran well

    c. would have run well

    d. ran more well

16. "Where does the sun go during the _____ asked little Kathy.

    a. night,"

    b. night"?,

    c. night,?"

    d. night?"

17. Choose the correct spelling.

    a. conscentious

    b. conscientios

    c. conscientious

    d. consceintious

18. I have finished studying for today.

What type of sentence is this?

    a. Imperative

    b. Interrogative

    c. Exclamatory

    d. Declarative

19. Which of the following sentences contains a redundant phrase?

    a. I haven't seen her for ages.

    b. My suitcase is books all the way to Amsterdam.

    c. The end result was very disappointing.

    d. None of the above.

20. Choose the correct sentence.

a. Their only employee with a nose ring is a young man named Daniel.

b. Their only employee is a young man named Daniel with a nose ring.

c. Their only employee is a young man with a nose ring named Daniel.

d. A and C are correct.

21. Choose the sentence with the correct grammar.

a. Everyone are to wear a black tie.

b. Everyone have to wear a black tie.

c. Everyone has to wear a black tie.

d. None of the above.

22. Choose the correct spelling.

a. leisuire

b. lesure

c. lesure

d. leisure

23. Choose the correct spelling.

a. pigeone

b. pigoen

c. pigeon

d. pidgeon

24. Choose the correct spelling.

a. odyessy

b. odeyssey

c. odysey

d. odyssey

25. Choose the sentence with the correct grammar.

    a. The salmon has been cooked.

    b. The salmon have been cooked.

    c. Both of the above.

    d. None of the above.

26. This is absolutely incredible _____

    a. !

    b. .

    c. :

    d. ;

27. Watch out for the broken glass _____

    a. .

    b. ?

    c. ,

    d. !

28. I still don't know exactly. That isn't _____ evidence.

    a. Undeterred

    b. Unrelenting

    c. Unfortunate

    d. Conclusive

29. He walked all the way downtown.

What is the simple subject of this sentence?

    a. He

    b. Walked

    c. Downtown

    d. All the way

30. He could manipulate the coins in his fingers very

    a. Brazenly

    b. Eloquently

    c. Boisterously

    d. Deftly

Section IV – Science

1. Which of the following is not true

    a. Genotypes are inherited information

    b. Phenotypes are inherited information

    c. Phenotypes are observed behavior

    d. Phenotypes include an organisms development

2. Electrons play a critical role in

    a. Electricity

    b. Magnetism

    c. Thermal conductivity

    d. All of the above

3. An idea concerning a phenomena and possible explanations for that phenomena is a/an

    a. Theory

    b. Experiment

    c. Inference

    d. Hypothesis

4. Define chromosomes.

a. Structures in a cell nucleus that carry genetic material.

b. Consist of thousands of DNA strands.

c. Total 46 in a normal human cell.

d. All of the above

5. What is one of the best known disorders that attack the immune system?

a. Rabies

b. HIV

c. Lung cancer

d. Muscular dystrophy

6. Which disease of the circulatory system is one of the most frequent causes of death in North America?

a. The cold

b. Pneumonia

c. Arthritis

d. Heart disease

7. Which of the following describes a plasma membrane?

a. Lipids with embedded proteins

b. An outer lipid layer and an inner lipid layer

c. Proteins embedded in lipid bilayer

d. Altering protein and lipid layers

8. What is the difference between Strong Nuclear Force and Weak Nuclear Force?

a. The Strong Nuclear Force is an attractive force that binds protons and neutrons and maintains the structure of the nucleus, and the Weak Nuclear Force is responsible for the radioactive beta decay and other subatomic reactions.

b. The Strong Nuclear Force is responsible for the radioactive beta decay and other subatomic reactions, and the Weak Nuclear Force is an attractive force that binds protons and neutrons and maintains the structure of the nucleus.

c. The Weak Nuclear Force is feeble and the Strong Nuclear Force is robust.

d. The Strong Nuclear Force is a negative force that releases protons and neutrons and threatens the structure of the nucleus, and the Weak Nuclear Force is an attractive force that binds protons and neutrons and maintains the structure of the nucleus.

9. What type of research studies the quality, type or components of a group, substance, or mixture?

a. Quantitative

b. Dependent

c. Scientific

d. Qualitative

10. Adaptation is

a. A trait that has evolved by natural selection.

b. A trait that has been bred by artificial selection.

c. A trait that has no function in an organism.

d. None of the above.

11. Describe a pH indicator.

a. A pH indicator measures hydrogen ions in a solution and show pH on a color scale.

b. A pH indicator measures oxygen ions in a solution and show pH on a color scale.

c. A pH indicator many different types of ions in a solution and shows pH on a color scale.

d. None of the above.

12. What is the earth's primary source of energy?

a. Water

b. The sun

c. Electromagnetic radiation

d. Weak nuclear force

13. What type of research is to determine the relationship between one thing (an independent variable) and another (a dependent or outcome variable) in a population?

a. Qualitative

b. Quantitative

c. Independent

d. Scientific

14. What can accept a hydrogen ion and can react with fats to form soaps?

a. Acid

b. Salt

c. Base

d. Foundation

15. Which gene, whose presence as a single copy, controls the expression of a trait?

    a. Principal gene

    b. Latent gene

    c. Recessive gene

    d. Dominant gene

16. Within taxonomy, plants and animals are considered two basic

    a. Families

    b. Kingdoms

    c. Domains

    d. Genus

17. Organisms grouped into the _____ Kingdom include all unicellular organisms lacking a definite cellular arrangement such as _____ and _____.

    a. Fungi, bacteria, algae

    b. Protista, bacteria, amphibian

    c. Protista, bacteria, algae

    d. Plantae, bacteria, algae

18. What is a common digestive affliction most people suffer at one time or other?

    a. Stomach cancer

    b. Ulceritis

    c. Indigestion

    d. The flu

19. What are the biochemical and biophysical activities that all living systems must be able to carry out to maintain life?

    a. Life sequences

    b. Life expectancies

    c. Life cycles

    d. Life functions

20. What disease of the circulatory system is often mistaken for a heart attack?

    a. Cardiac arrest

    b. High blood pressure

    c. Angina

    d. Acid reflux

21. Define a biological class.

    a. A collection of similar or like living entities.

    b. Two or more animals in a group, all having the same parent.

    c. All animals sharing the same living environment.

    d. All plant life that share the same physical properties.

22. What type of foods that stay in the stomach the longest?

    a. Fats

    b. Proteins

    c. Carbohydrates

    d. Vitamins

23. What is a graphical description of feeding relation-ships among species in an ecological community?

    a. Food web

    b. Food chain

    c. Food network

    d. Food sequence

24. What is the diagram that is used to predict an out-come of a particular cross or breeding experiment?

    a. Genetic puzzle

    b. Genome project

    c. Hybrid theorem

    d. Punnett square

25. Which, if any, of the following statements about pro-karyotic cells is false?

    a. Prokaryotic cells include such organisms as E. coli and Streptococcus.

    b. Prokaryotic cells lack internal membranes and organ-elles.

    c. Prokaryotic cells break down food using cellular res-piration and fermentation.

    d. All of these statements are true.

26. What is the process of converting observed phenomena into data is called?

    a. Calculation

    b. Measurement

    c. Valuation

    d. Estimation

27. The mass number of an atom is

a. The total number of particles that make it up.

b. The total weight of an atom.

c. The total mass of an atom.

d. None of the above.

28. What is sublimation?

a. A phase transition from liquid to gas.

b. A phase transition from solid to gas.

c. A phase transition from gas to liquid.

d. A phase transition from gas to solid.

29. How is exhalation accomplished?

a. By the abdominal muscles

b. By the chest muscles

c. By the esophagus

d. By the nasal passageway

30. What three processes are involved in cell division of Eukaryotic cells?

a. Meiosis, mitosis, and interphase

b. Meiosis, mitosis, and interphase

c. Mitosis, kinematisis, and interphase

d. Mitosis, cytokinesis, and interphase

31. Describe genotypes.

a. The genetic makeup, as distinguished from the physical appearance, of an organism or a group of organisms.

b. The combination of alleles located on homologous chromosomes that determines a specific characteristic or trait.

c. Is the inheritable information carried by all living organisms.

d. All of the above.

32. What does the respiratory system primarily oxygenate?

a. The brain

b. The limbs

c. The heart

d. The blood

33. What chain of nucleotides plays an important role in the creation of new proteins?

a. Deoxyribonucleic acid (DNA) is a chain of nucleotides that plays an important role in the creation of new proteins.

b. Ribonucleic acid (RNA) is a chain of nucleotides that plays an important role in the creation of new proteins.

c. There are no chains of nucleotides that play a role in the creation of proteins.

d. None of the above.

34. A practical test designed with the intention that its results will be relevant to a particular theory or set of theories is a/an

    a. Experiment

    b. Practicum

    c. Theory

    d. Design

35. Strong chemical bonds include

    a. Dipole - dipole interactions.

    b. Hydrogen bonding.

    c. Covalent or ionic bonds.

    d. None of the above.

36. What is the process that the immune system adapts over time to be more efficient in recognizing pathogens?

    a. Acquired immunity

    b. AIDS

    c. Pathogens

    d. Acquired deficiency

37. What is a group of tissues that perform a specific function or group of functions?

    a. System

    b. Tissue

    c. Group

    d. Organ

38. What is the measure of an experiment's ability to yield the same or compatible results in different clinical experiments or statistical trials?

    a. Variability

    b. Validity

    c. Control measure

    d. Reliability

39. Describe each chemical element in the periodic table.

    a. Each chemical element has a unique atomic number representing the number of electrons in its nucleus.

    b. Each chemical element has a varying atomic number depending on the number of protons in its nucleus.

    c. Each chemical element has a unique atomic number representing the number of protons in its nucleus.

    d. None of the above.

40. The immune system is

    a. The system that expels waste from the body.

    b. The system that expels carbon dioxide from the body.

    c. The system that protects the body from disease and infection.

    d. The system that circulates blood through the body.

41. The binding membrane of an animal cell is called

    a. The biological membrane.

    b. The cell coat.

    c. The unit membrane.

    d. The plasma membrane.

42. Define organelles.

a. A protein in a cell

b. An enzyme in a cell

c. A specialized subunit of a cell with a specific function

d. A cell membrane

43. A solution with a pH value of less than 7 is

a. Acid solution.

b. Base solution.

c. Neutral pH solution.

d. None of the above.

44. Is a catalyst changed by a reaction?

a. Yes

b. No

c. It may be changed depending on the other chemicals.

45. What is the prediction that an observed difference is due to chance alone and not due to a systematic cause? This hypothesis is tested by statistical analysis, and either accepted or rejected.

a. Null hypothesis

b. Hypothesis

c. Control

d. Variable

46. In science, industry, and statistics, the _____ of a measurement system is the degree of closeness of measurements of a quantity to its actual (true) value.

    a. Mistake
    b. Uncertainty
    c. Accuracy
    d. Error

47. What is a more common name for the circulatory system disease known as hypertension?

    a. Anemia
    b. High blood pressure
    c. Angina
    d. Cardiac arrest

48. Given a normal distribution, what is the difference between the maximum value and the minimum value?

    a. Distribution
    b. Range
    c. Mode
    d. Median

Quick Reference Answer Key

Part I - Reading

1. B
2. C
3. A
4. A
5. A
6. B
7. C
8. A
9. B
10. A
11. B
12. A
13. B
14. B
15. D
16. A
17. A
18. B
19. C
20. C
21. D
22. C
23. B
24. C
25. A
26. D
27. B
28. B
29. C
30. D
31. B
32. C
33. C
34. A
35. B
36. C
37. B
38. A

39. A
40. C
41. A
42. A

Section II – Math

1. D
2. A
3. C
4. B
5. A
6. D
7. A
8. D
9. D
10. A
11. C
12. C
13. C
14. C
15. A
16. A
17. D
18. D
19. A
20. C
21. A
22. A
23. C
24. D
25. B
26. D
27. B
28. A
29. A
30. A

Section III – English and Language Usage

1. D
2. A
3. A
4. B
5. A
6. A
7. A
8. D
9. C
10. A
11. C
12. B
13. C
14. C
15. B
16. D
17. C
18. D
19. C
20. D
21. C
22. D
23. C
24. D
25. C
26. A
27. D
28. D
29. A
30. D

Section IV – Science

1. B
2. D
3. D
4. D

5. B
6. D
7. C
8. A
9. D
10. A
11. A
12. B
13. B
14. C
15. D
16. B
17. C
18. C
19. D
20. C
21. A
22. A
23. A
24. D
25. D
26. B
27. A
28. B
29. A
30. D
31. D
32. D
33. B
34. A
35. C
36. A
37. D
38. D
39. C
40. C
41. D
42. C
43. A
44. B
45. A
46. C
47. B
48. B

Answer Key with Explanations

1. B
We can infer an important part of the respiratory system are the lungs. From the passage, "Molecules of oxygen and carbon dioxide are passively exchanged, by diffusion, between the gaseous external environment and the blood. This exchange process occurs in the alveolar region of the lungs."

Therefore, one primary function for the respiratory system is the exchange of oxygen and carbon dioxide, and this process occurs in the lungs. We can therefore infer that the lungs are an important part of the respiratory system.

2. C
The process by which molecules of oxygen and carbon dioxide are passively exchanged is diffusion.

This is a definition type question. Scan the passage for references to "oxygen," "carbon dioxide," or "exchanged."

3. A
The organ that plays an important role in gas exchange in amphibians is the skin.

Scan the passage for references to "amphibians," and find the answer.

4. A
The three physiological zones of the respiratory system are Conducting, transitional, respiratory zones.

5. A
Secede most nearly means to break away from because the 11 states wanted to leave the United States and form their own country.

Choice B is incorrect because the states were not accomplishing anything
Choice C is incorrect because the states were trying to leave the USA not join it. Choice D is incorrect because the states seceded before they lost the war.

6. B
Look at the dates in the passage. The shots were fired on April 12 and Congress declared war on April 14.

Choice A is incorrect because the dates show clearly which happened first. Choice C is incorrect because the passage states that Lincoln was against slavery. Choice D is incorrect because it never mentions who was or was not at Fort Sumter.

7. C
The passage clearly states that Lee surrendered to Grant after the capture of the capital of the Confederacy, which is Richmond.
Choice A is incorrect because the war continued for 2 years after Gettysburg.

Choice B is incorrect because that battle is never mentioned in the passage. Choice
D is incorrect because the capture of the capital occurred after the march to the sea.

8. A
When the passage said that the North had abolished slavery, it implies that slaves were no longer allowed to be had in the North. In essence slavery was banned.

Choice B is incorrect because it makes no sense relative to the context of the passage. Choice C is incorrect because we know the North was fighting slavery, not for it. Choice D is incorrect because slavery is not a tangible thing that can be destroyed. It is a practice that had to be outlawed or banned.

9. B
The first paragraph tells us that myths are a true account of the remote past.

The second paragraph tells us that, "myths generally take place during a primordial age, when the world was still young, before achieving its current form."

Putting these two together, we can infer that humankind used myth to explain how the world was created.

10. A
This passage is about different types of stories. First, the passage explains myths, and then compares other types of stories to myths.

11. B
From the passage, "Unlike myths, folktales can take place at any time and any place, and the natives do not usually consider them true or sacred."

12. A
Based on the partial table of contents, this book is most likely about how to answer multiple choice.

13. B
This passage describes the different categories for traditional stories. The other choices are facts from the passage, not the main idea of the passage. The main idea of a passage will always be the most general statement. For example, choice A, Myths, fables, and folktales are not the same thing, and each describes a specific type of story. This is a true statement from the passage, but not the main idea of the passage, since the passage also talks about how some cultures may classify a story as a myth and others as a folktale.

The statement, from choice B, Traditional stories can be categorized in different ways by different people, is a more general statement that describes the passage.

14. B
Choice B is the best choice, categories that group traditional stories according to certain characteristics.

Choices A and C are false and can be eliminated right away. Choice D is designed to confuse. Choice D may be true, but it is not mentioned in the passage.

15. D
The best answer is D, traditional stories themselves are a part of the larger category of folklore, which may also include costumes, gestures, and music.

All the other choices are false. Traditional stories are part of the larger category of Folklore, which includes other things, not the other way around.

16. A
There is a distinct difference between a myth and a legend, both are folktales.

17. A
Victoria is about 5 miles from Burnaby.

18. B
The Village Hall is about 5 miles from Victoria.

19. C
To be infamous means to be remembered for an evil or terrible action. Therefore, the word infamy means to remember a bad or terrible thing.

Choice A is incorrect because being famous is not the same as being infamous. Choice D is incorrect because Pearl Harbor was not forgotten.

20. C
Each other answer set contains the name of at least one country who was not part of the AXIS powers.

21. D
The answer is stated directly in the passage.

Choice A is in correct because there was no indication that Japan would attack San Diego. Choice B is incorrect because the attack on Pearl Harbor was a surprise. Choice C is incorrect because Roosevelt was not planning to attack Japan.

22. C
The passage clearly states that Japan planned a surprise attack. They chose that early time to catch the U.S. military off guard. Choice A is incorrect because the military does not sleep late. Choice B is incorrect because there is no law against bombing countries. Choice D is incorrect because it makes no sense.

23. B

This question tests the reader's summarization skills. Choice A is a very broad statement that may or may not be true, and seems to be in context, but has nothing to do with the passage. The author does mention that the statue was probably used on a temple dedicated to the Greek gods (D), but in no way discusses or argues for the gods' attitude toward or claim on these temples or its faucets. Nike does indeed lead the gods into a war (the Titan war), as choice C suggests, but this is not mentioned by the passage and students who know this may be drawn to this answer but have not done a close enough analysis of the text that is actually in the passage. Choice B is appropriately expository, and connects the titular emphasis to the idea that the Greek gods are very important to Greek culture.

24. C
This question tests the reader's summarization skills. The test for question choice C is pulled straight from the paragraph, but is not word for word, so it may seem too obvious to be the right answer. The passage does talk about Nike being the goddess of war, as choice A states, but the third paragraph only touches on it and it is an inference that soldiers destroyed the statue, when this question is asking specifically for what the third paragraph actually stated. Choice B is also straight from the text, with a minor but key change: the inclusion of the words "all" and "never" are too limiting and the passage does not suggest that these limits exist. If a reader selects choice D, they are also making an inference that is misguided for this type of question. The paragraph does state that the arms and head are "lost" but does not suggest who lost them.

25. A
This question tests the reader's ability to recognize function in writing. Choice B can be eliminated based on the purpose of the passage, which is expository and not persuasive. The author may or may not feel this way, but the passage does not show evidence of being argumentative for that purpose. Choices C and D are both details found in the text, neither of them encompasses the entire message of the passage, which has an overall message of learning about culture from art and making guesses about how the two are related, as suggested by choice A.

26. D
This question tests the reader's ability to understand function within writing. Most of the possible selections are very general statements which may or may not be true. It probably is a student who is taking the test on which this question is featured (A), but the author makes no address to the test taker and is not talking to the audience in terms of the test. Likewise, it may also be true that students read more than adults (C), mandated by schools and grades, but the focus on the verb "read" in the first sentence is too narrow and misses the larger purpose of the passage; the same could be said for choice B. While all the statements could be true, choice D is the most germane, and infers the purpose of the passage without making assumptions that could be incorrect.

27. B
The time limit for radar detectors is 14 days. Since you made the purchase 15 days ago, you do not qualify for the guarantee.

28. B
Since you made the purchase 10 days ago, you are covered by the guarantee. Since it is an advertised price at a different store, ABC Electric will "beat" the price by 10% of the difference, which is,

500 – 400 = 100 – difference in price

100 X 10% = $10 – 10% of the difference

The advertised lower price is $400. ABC will beat this price by 10% so they will refund $100 + 10 = $110.

29. C
The purpose of this passage is to persuade.

30. D
This question tests the reader's summarization skills. The question is asking very generally about the message of the passage, and the title, "Ways Characters Communicate in Theater," is one indication of that. The other choices A, B, and C are all directly from the text, and therefore readers may be inclined to select one of them, but are too specific to

encapsulate the entirety of the passage and its message.

31. B

The paragraph on soliloquies mentions "To be or not to be," and it is from the context of that paragraph that readers may understand that because "To be or not to be" is a soliloquy, Hamlet will be introspective, or thoughtful, while delivering it. It is true that actors deliver soliloquies alone, and may be "solitary" (A), but "thoughtful" (B) is more true to the overall idea of the paragraph. Readers may choose choice C because drama and theater can be used interchangeably and the passage mentions that soliloquies are unique to theater (and therefore drama), but this answer is not specific enough to the paragraph in question. Readers may pick up on the theme of life and death and Hamlet's true intentions and select that he is "hopeless" (D), but those themes are not discussed either by this paragraph or passage, as a close textual reading and analysis confirms.

32. C

This question tests the reader's grammatical skills. Choice B seems logical, but parenthesis are actually considered to be a stronger break in a sentence than commas are, and along this line of thinking, actually disrupt the sentence more. Choices A and D make comparisons between theater and film that are simply not made in the passage, and may or may not be true. This detail does clarify the statement that asides are most unique to theater by adding that it is not completely unique to theater, which may have been why the author didn't chose not to delete it and instead used parentheses to designate the detail's importance (C).

33. C

This question tests the reader's vocabulary and contextualization skills. A may or may not be true, but focuses on the wrong function of the word "give" and ignores the rest of the sentence, which is more relevant to what the passage is discussing. Choices B and D may also be selected if the reader depends too literally on the word "give," failing to grasp the more abstract function of the word that is the focus of choice C, which also properly acknowledges the entirety of the passage and its meaning.

34. A
We can infer that an important purpose of the circulatory system is that of fighting diseases.

35. B
Humans have a closed circulatory system.

36. C
Besides blood, the heart and the blood vessels form the cardiovascular system.

37. B
The digestive system, along with the circulatory system, helps provide nutrients to keep the human heart pumping.

38. A
We can infer that blood is responsible for transporting oxygen to the cells.

39. A
Human blood cells suspended in plasma.

40. C
Calcium is not contained in blood plasma.

From the passage, "[Blood Plasma] contains dissolved proteins, glucose, mineral ions, hormones, carbon dioxide, platelets and the blood cells themselves."

41. A
The lungs exhale the carbon dioxide after venous blood has been carried from body tissues.

42. A
The main idea of this passage is that the human skeleton is an important and complicated system of the body.

We can infer the skeleton is important because it protects important organs like brain, lungs and heart. We know the skeleton is complicated because it consists of several parts, (ligaments, tendons, muscles and cartilage) and 206 bones.

This general statement best describes the passage. The other choices are details mentioned in the passage.

Section II – Math

1. D
We understand that each of the n employees earn s amount of salary weekly. This means that one employee earns s salary weekly. So; Richard has ns amount of money to employ n employees for a week.

We are asked to find the number of days n employees can be employed with x amount of money. We can do simple direct proportion:

If Richard can employ n employees for 7 days with ns amount of money,

   Richard can employ n employees for y days with x amount of money ... y is the number of days we need to find.

We can do cross multiplication:

$y = (x \cdot 7)/(ns)$

$y = 7x/ns$

2. A
Five greater than 3 times a number.
5 + 3 times a number.
$3X + 5$

3. C
MMXIII is 2013. $1,000 + 1,000 + 10 + 1 + 1 + 1.$

4. B
$5b + 21 = 66$, $5b = 66 - 21 = 45$, $5b = 45$, $b = 45/5 = 9$

5. A
The number is 51.738. The last digit, in the 1,000th place, 2, is less than 5, so it is discarded. Answer = 765.368.

6. D
This is a simple direct proportion problem:
If Lynn can type 1 page in p minutes, she can type x pages in 5 minutes

We do cross multiplication: x•p = 5•1

Then,

x = 5/p

7. A
This is an inverse ration problem.

1/x = 1/a + 1/b where a is the time Sally can paint a house, b is the time John can paint a house, x is the time Sally and John can together paint a house.

So,

1/x = 1/4 + 1/6 ... We use the least common multiple in the denominator that is 24:

1/x = 6/24 + 4/24

1/x = 10/24

x = 24/10

x = 2.4 hours.

In other words; 2 hours + 0.4 hours = 2 hours + 0.4•60 minutes

= 2 hours 24 minutes

8. D
The cost of the dishwasher = $450

15% discount amount = 450•15/100 = $67.5

The discounted price = 450 − 67.5 = $382.5

20% additional discount amount on lowest price = 382.5•20/100 = $76.5

So, the final discounted price = 382.5 - 76.5 = $306.00

9. D
Original price = x,
80/100 = 12590/X,

80X = 1259000,
X = 15,737.50.

10. A
25% = 25/100 = 1/4

11. C
125/100 = 1.25

12. C
24/56 = 3/7 (divide numerator and denominator by 8)

13. C
Converting a fraction into a decimal – divide the numerator by the denominator – so 71/1000 = .071. Dividing by 1000 moves the decimal point 3 places to the left.

14. C
9 is in the ten thousandths place in 1.7389, which is 4 places to the right of the decimal point.

15. A
(6-4) (3/5 – 4/5) = 2 (3-4/5) = since 3 is less than 4, we would have to subtract 1 from the whole number besides the fraction, therefore 1 4/5

16. A
Step 1: Set up the formula to calculate the dose to be given in mg as per weight of the child:-
Dose ordered X Weight in Kg = Dose to be given
Step 2: 100 mg X 23 kg = 2300 mg
(Convert 50 lb to Kg, 1 lb = 0.4536 kg, hence 50 lb = 50 X 0.4536 = 22.68 kg approx. 23 kg)
2300 mg/230 mg X 1 tablet/1 = 2300/230 = 10 tablets

17. D
To find the total turnout in all three polling stations, we need to proportion the number of voters to the number of all registered voters.

Number of total voters = 945 + 860 + 1210 = 3015

Number of total registered voters = 1270 + 1050 + 1440 =

3760

Percentage turnout over all three polling stations =
3015•100/3760 = 80.19%

Checking the answers, we round 80.19 to the nearest whole
number: 80%

18. D
600 mg/ 200 mg X 1 tablet/1 = 600/200 = 3 tablets

19. A
At 100% efficiency 1 machine produces 1450/10 = 145 m of
cloth.

At 95% efficiency, 4 machines produce 4•145•95/100 = 551
m of cloth.

At 90% efficiency, 6 machines produce 6•145•90/100 = 783
m of cloth.

Total cloth produced by all 10 machines = 551 + 783 = 1334
m

Since the information provided and the question are based
on 8 hours, we did not need to use time to reach the answer.

20. C
1 foot = 12 inches, 60 feet = 60 x 12 = 720 inches.

21. A
The ratio between black and blue pens is 7 to 28 or 7:28.
Bring to the lowest terms by dividing both sides by 7 gives
1:4.

22. A
1 millimeter = 10 centimeter, 100 millimeter = 100/10 = 10
centimeters.

23. C
1 gallon = 4 quarts, 3 gallons = 3 x 4 = 12 quarts.

24. D
1 inch on map = 2,000 inches on ground. So, 5.2 inches on

map = 5.2•2,000 = 10,400 inches on ground.

25. B
There are 1000 ml in a liter. 0.05/1000 = 0.00005 liters.

26. D
X% of 120 = 30,
X/100 = 30/120
So X = 30/120 x 100/1
3000/120 = 300/12
X = 25

27. B
There are 52 cards in total. Smith has 16 cards in which he can win. Therefore, his probability of winning in a single game will be 16/52. Simon has 20 winning cards so his probability of winning in single draw is 20/52.

28. A
There are 100 centimeters in a meter, so 100 X .45 meters = 45.

29. A
Based on this graph, a person that is 85 or older will make 26.2 visits to the hospital every year.

30. A
A person aged 95 or older would make 31.3 or more visits.

Section III – English and Language Usage

1. D
The preposition "to" is correct. 'To' here means give.

2. A
"Lie" means to recline, and does not take an object. "lay" means to place and does take an object.

3. A
Past unreal conditional. Takes the form,

[If ... Past Perfect ...., ... would have + past participle ...]

4. B
This sentence is in the present tense, so "to find" is correct.

5. A
Always use the singular verb form for nouns like politics, wages, mathematics, innings, news, advice, summons, furniture, information, poetry, machinery, vacation, scenery etc.

6. A
Possessive pronouns ending in 's' take an apostrophe before the 's': one's; everyone's; somebody's, nobody else's, etc.

7. A
A bonus is an extra feature, so added is redundant.

8. D
When talking about something that didn't happen in the past, use the past perfect (if I had done).

9. C
"Lie" means to recline, and does not take an object. "Lay" means to place and does take an object. Peter lay the books on the table (the books are the direct object), or the telephone poles were lying on the road (no direct object).

10. A
Titles of short stories are enclosed in quotation marks.

11. C
No additional punctuation is required here.

12. B
Here the word "sale" is used as a "word" and not as a word in the sentence, so quotation marks are used.

13. C
If one of the subjects linked by "either," "or,""nor" or "neither" is in plural form, then the verb should also be in plural, and the verb should be close to the plural subject.

14. C
Titles of short stories are enclosed in quotation marks, and commas always go inside quotation marks.

15. B
"Ran well" is correct. "Ran good" is never correct.

16. D
Commas and periods always go inside quotation marks. Question marks that are part of a quote also go inside quotation marks; however, if the writer quotes a statement as part of a larger question, the question mark is placed after the quotation mark.

17. C
Conscientious is the correct spelling.

18. D
This is a declarative sentence.

19. C
A result is something that occurs at the end, so an 'end result' is redundant.

20. D
Both A and C are correct.

> a. Their only employee with a nose ring is a young man named Daniel.
>
> c. Their only employee is a young man with a nose ring named Daniel.

21. C
Use a singular verb with either, each, neither, everyone and many.

22. D
Leisure is the correct spelling.

23. C
Pigeon is the correct spelling.

24. D
Odyssey is the correct spelling.

25. C
Nouns like deer, sheep, swine, salmon etc can take a singular or plural verb depending if they are used in their singular

or plural form.
26. A
Use an exclamation mark to end an exclamatory sentence, that is, at the end of a statement showing strong emotion.

27. D
Use an exclamation mark after an imperative sentence if the command is urgent and forceful.

28. D
Conclusive ADJECTIVE providing an end to something; decisive.

29. A
'He' is the simple subject of this sentence.

30. D
Deftly: VERB. Quick and skillful.

Section IV – Science

1. B
The only statement that is NOT true is, Phenotypes are inherited information.

2. D
All the above are true. Electrons play an essential role in electricity, magnetism, and thermal conductivity.

3. D
An idea concerning a phenomena and possible explanations for that phenomena is an hypothesis.

4. D
All of the above
a. Structures in a cell nucleus that carry genetic material.
b. Consist of one very long strand of DNA
c. Total 46 in a normal human cell.

5. B
One of the best known disorders that attack the immune
system is HIV (the virus that causes AIDS).

6. D
The circulatory system disease that is one of the most frequent causes of death in North America is heart disease.

7. C
The plasma membrane or cell membrane protects the cell
from outside forces. It consists of the lipid bilayer with embedded proteins.

8. A
The Strong Nuclear Force is an attractive force that binds
protons and neutrons and maintains the structure of the
nucleus, and the Weak Nuclear Force is responsible for the
radioactive beta decay and other subatomic reactions.

Note: The Weak Nuclear Force is so named because it is
only effective for short distances. Nevertheless, it is through
the Weak Nuclear Force that the sun provides us with energy by allowing one element to change into another element. [23]

9. D
Qualitative research deals with the quality, type or components of a group, substance, or mixture.

10. A
Adaptation is a trait that has evolved by natural selection.

11. A
A pH indicator measures hydrogen ions in a solution and
show pH on a color scale.

12. B
The sun is the earth's primary source of energy.

13. B
The goal of quantitative research is to determine the rela-

tionship between one thing (an independent variable) and another (a dependent or outcome variable) in a population.

14. C
A base is any substance that can accept a hydrogen ion and can react with fats to form soaps.

15. D
The dominant gene controls the expression of a trait.

16. B
Plants and animals are Kingdoms. There are six recognized kingdoms: Animalia, Plantae, Protista, Fungi, Bacteria, and Archaea.

17. C
Organisms grouped into the **Protista** Kingdom include all unicellular organisms lacking a definite cellular arrangement such as **bacteria** and **algae.**

18. C
Indigestion is a common digestive affliction that most people suffer at one time or other.

19. D
Life functions are the biochemical and biophysical activities that all living systems must be able to carry out to maintain life.

20. C
Angina is frequently mistaken for a heart attack. Angina pectoris, commonly known as angina, is severe chest pain due to ischemia (a lack of blood, thus a lack of oxygen supply) of the heart muscle, generally due to obstruction or spasm of the coronary arteries (the heart's blood vessels). [24]

21. A
A collection of similar or like living entities. Class has the same meaning in biology as rank. Common classes or ranks include species, order, and phylum.

22. A
Fats stay in the stomach the longest.

23. A
A food web is a graphical description of feeding relationships among species in an ecological community.

Note: A food web differs from a food chain in that the latter shows only a portion of the food web involving a simple, linear series of species (e.g., predator, herbivore, plant) connected by feeding links. A food web aims to depict a more complete picture of the feeding relationships, and can be considered a bundle of many interconnected food chains occurring within the community.

24. D
A Punnett square resembles a game of tic-tac-toe, in which the genotypes of the parents gametes are entered first, so that subsequent combinations can be calculated.

25. D
All of these statements are true.

> a. Prokaryotic cells include such organisms as E. coli and Streptococcus.
>
> b. Prokaryotic cells lack internal membranes and organelles.
>
> c. Prokaryotic cells break down food using cellular respiration and fermentation.

26. B
The process of converting observed phenomena into data is called Measurement.

27. A
The mass number of an atom is the total number of particles (protons and neutrons) that make it up.

28. B
Sublimation is the direct phase transition from solid to gas.

29. A
Exhalation is often accomplished by the abdominal muscles.

30. D
In Eukaryotic cells, the cell cycle is the cycle of events involving cell division, including mitosis, cytokinesis, and interphase.

31. D
All of the choices are correct.

> a. The genetic makeup, as distinguished from the physical appearance, of an organism or a group of organisms.
>
> b. The combination of alleles located on homologous chromosomes that determines a specific characteristic or trait.
>
> c. Is the inheritable information carried by all living organisms.

32. D
The blood is the primarily oxygenated through the work of the respiratory system.

33. B
Ribonucleic acid (RNA) is a chain of nucleotides that play an important role in the creation of new proteins.

34. A
A practical test designed with the intention that its results will be relevant to a particular theory or set of theories is an experiment.

35. C
Covalent or ionic bonds are considered "strong bonds."

36. A
The process by which the immune system adapts over time to be more efficient in recognizing pathogens is known as acquired immunity.

37. D
An organ is a group of tissues that perform a specific function or group of functions.

38. D
Reliability refers to the measure of an experiment's ability to yield the same or compatible results in different clinical experiments or statistical trials.

39. C
Each chemical element has a unique atomic number representing the number of protons in its nucleus.

40. C
The immune system is the system that protects the body from disease and infection.

41. D
The plasma membrane surrounds the cell and functions as an interface between the living interior of the cell and the nonliving exterior. [19]

42. C
An organelle is a specialized subunit of a cell with a specific function.

43. A
A solution with a pH value of less than 7 is acid. A pH value of 7 is neutral.

44. B
A catalyst is never changed in a chemical reaction.

45. A
The prediction that an observed difference is due to chance alone and not due to a systematic cause; statistical analysis tested this hypothesis, and it is accepted or rejected is the **null hypothesis**.

46. C
In science and engineering, the Accuracy of a measurement

system is the degree of closeness of measurements of a quantity to its actual (true) value.

47. B
High blood pressure is a more common name for the circulatory system disease known as hypertension. Hypertension (HTN) or high blood pressure is a cardiac chronic medical condition in which the systemic arterial blood pressure is elevated.

48. B
The range of a distribution is the difference between the maximum value and the minimum value.

Conclusion

CONGRATULATIONS! You have made it this far because you have applied yourself diligently to practicing for the exam and no doubt improved your potential score considerably! Getting into a good school is a huge step in a journey that might be challenging at times but will be many times more rewarding and fulfilling. That is why being prepared is so important.

Study then Practice and then Succeed!

Good Luck!

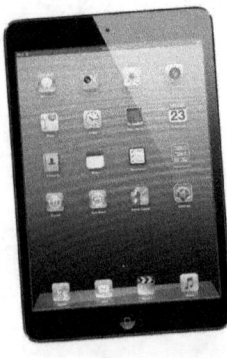

FREE Ebook Version

Go to **http://tinyurl.com/m4abcfa**

Register for Free Updates and More Practice Test Questions

Register your purchase at www.test-preparation.ca/register.html for fast and convenient access to updates, errata, free test tips and more practice test questions.

HOBET Test Strategy!

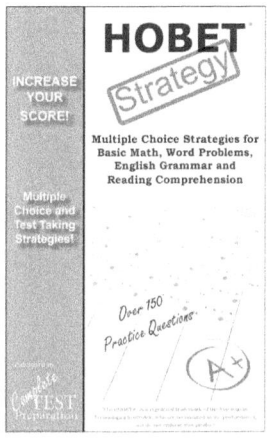

Learn to increase your score using time-tested secrets for answering multiple choice questions! |

This practice book has everything you need to know about answering multiple choice questions on a standardized test!

You will learn 12 strategies for answering multiple choice questions and then practice each strategy with over 45 reading comprehension multiple choice questions, with extensive commentary from exam experts!

Maybe you have read this kind of thing before, and maybe feel you don't need it, and you are not sure if you are going to buy this Book.

Remember though, it only a few percentage points divide the PASS from the FAIL students.

Even if our multiple choice strategies increase your score by a few percentage points, isn't that worth it?

https://www.createspace.com/4170757
Enter Code PKEMHHT4 for 25% off!

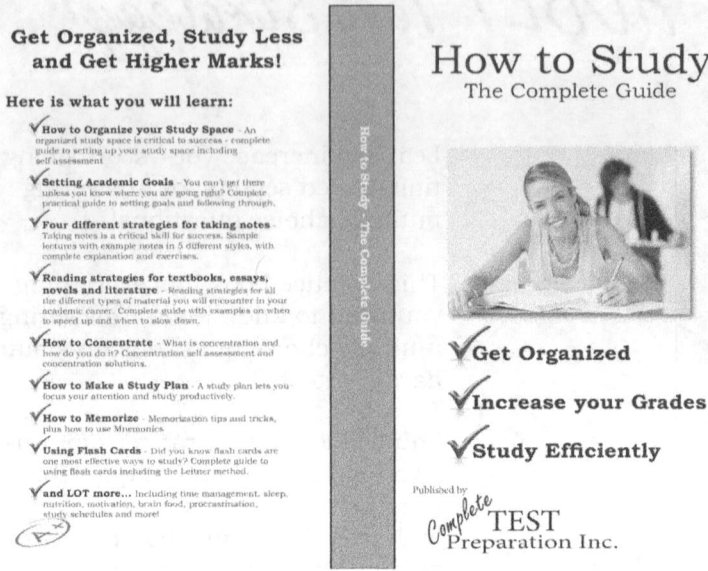

Get Organized, Study Less and Get Higher Marks!

Here is what you will learn:

- How to Organize your Study Space

- Four different strategies for taking notes

- Reading strategies for textbooks, essays, novels and literature

- How to Concentrate - What is concentration and how do you do it!

- Using Flash Cards - Complete guide to using flash cards including the Leitner method.

and LOT more... Including time management, sleep, nutrition, motivation, brain food, procrastination, study schedules and more!

https://www.createspace.com/4060298

Enter Code LYFZGQB5 for 25% off!

NOTES

Modified portions of the text where noted below is used under the Creative Commons Attribution-ShareAlike 3.0 License

http://en.wikipedia.org/wiki/Wikipedia:Text_of_Creative_Commons_Attribution-ShareAlike_3.0_Unported_License

[1] Infection. In Wikipedia. Retrieved November 12, 2012 frohttp://en.wikipedia.org/wiki/Infection

[2] Thunderstorm. In *Wikipedia*. Retrieved November 12, 2010 from en.wikipedia.org/wiki/Thunderstorm.

[3] Meteorology. In *Wikipedia*. Retrieved November 12, 2010 from en.wikipedia.org/wiki/Outline_of_meteorology.

[4] U.S. Navy Seal. In *Wikipedia*. Retrieved November 12, 2010 from en.wikipedia.org/wiki/United_States_Navy_SEALs.

[5] Gardening. In *Wikipedia*. Retrieved January 2, 2012 from en.wikipedia.org/wiki/Gardening.

[6] What Causes DNA Mutations? (n.d.) Learn.Genetics. http://learn.genetics.utah.edu/archive/sloozeworm/mutationbg.html

[7] The Four Fundamental Forces. (n.d.) Oracle Education Foundation. Retrieved from http://library.thinkquest.org/27930/forces.htm

[8] Cell Membrane. In Wikipedia. Retrieved January 2, 2012 from http://en.wikipedia.org/wiki/Cell_membrane.

[9] Thoracic Diaphram. In Wikipedia. Retrieved January 2, 2012 from http://en.wikipedia.org/wiki/Thoracic_diaphragm.

[10] Respiratory System. In *Wikipedia*. Retrieved November 12, 2010 from en.wikipedia.org/wiki/Respiratory_system.

[11] Mythology. In *Wikipedia*. Retrieved November 12, 2010 from en.wikipedia.org/wiki/Mythology.

[12] Circulatory System. In *Wikipedia*. Retrieved November 12, 2010 from en.wikipedia.org/wiki/Circulatory_system

[13] Blood. In Wikipedia. Retrieved November 12,2010 from http://en.wikipedia.org/wiki/Blood.

[14] Human Skeleton. In Wikipedia. Retrieved November 12,2010 from http://en.wikipedia.org/wiki/Human_skeleton.

[15] The Four Fundamental Forces. (n.d.) Oracle Education Foundation. Retrieved from http://library.thinkquest.org/27930/forces.htm

[16] Angina. In Wikipedia. Retrieved January 20, 2013 from http://en.wikipedia.org/wiki/Angina.